CLINICAL PRACTICE
WITH INDIVIDUALS

CLINICAL PRACTICE WITH INDIVIDUALS

Mark A. Mattaini

NASW PRESS

National Association of Social Workers
Washington, DC

Jay J. Cayner, ACSW, LSW, *President*
Josephine Nieves, MSW, PhD, *Executive Director*

Linda Beebe, *Executive Editor*
Nancy Winchester, *Editorial Services Director*
Stephen D. Pazdan, *Project Manager*
Patricia D. Wolf, Wolf Publications, Inc., *Copy Editor*
Ronald W. Wolf, Wolf Publications, Inc., *Copy Editor*
Kathleen Savory, *Proofreader*
Beth Gyorgy, *Proofreader*
Robert Elwood, *Indexer*

Library of Congress Cataloging-in-Publication Data
Mattaini, Mark A.
   Clinical practice with individuals / Mark A. Mattaini.
     p.   cm.
   Includes bibliographical references (p.   ) and index.
   ISBN 0-87101-270-7 (alk. paper)
   1. Psychiatric social work.   2. Social case work.   I. Title.
HV689.M37   1996   96–42938
361.3'2—dc20   CIP

Printed in the United States of America

For those with the courage and integrity
to do social work,
especially CHM & CTL
<<< >>>

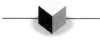

CONTENTS

INTRODUCTION

Professional social work seeks to enhance adaptations among clients and the systems within which they are embedded (Meyer, 1993). Many practice models exist to accomplish this. Behavioral and cognitive–behavioral approaches, the effectiveness of which is supported by extensive data, are among these practice models, and many excellent books, chapters, and articles presenting them have been written (Gambrill, in press; Granvold, 1994; Schwartz, 1983; Schwartz & Goldiamond, 1975; Thyer, Himle, & Santa, 1986).

So why is this book needed?

- There exists a lack of information that applies current state-of-the-art behavioral theory and findings from basic research (some of which have never, to my knowledge, been extended to applied work) to social work practice, even though we have learned a great deal in recent years. For example, cognitive approaches demonstrated their usefulness in the 1970s. Only recently, however, has it become clear that cognition can most usefully be viewed as a subset of behavior, which leads to a new understanding of why cognitive techniques work and how to apply them in practice in an organic way (Hayes, 1992; Kohlenberg & Tsai, 1991, 1994). Both behavioral and cognitive–behavioral strategies are outlined in this book but within an integrated conceptual framework.

- Much of what is available in the literature is not grounded firmly in the professional practice of social work. Many techniques are borrowed from other disciplines, and the principles of the science of behavior do not change depending on who is using them. Social workers, however, do something other than what psychologists or certified addictions counselors do. Social work practice is not a collection of unrelated techniques for changing the behavior of individuals but rather an integrated approach for enhancing the fit between client and environment. Ecobehavioral social work practice is not the same as what other professions do, but this fact has often not been emphasized, and perhaps sometimes not recognized, in the behavioral social work literature.

+ Because many of the most recent behavioral findings have so far been presented only at a highly technical level, the learning curve can be steep. Although an understanding of concepts such as differential reinforcement and equivalence relations is important to effective practice, most social workers do not yet speak that language. My goal in this book is to present practical guidelines for practice that are firmly rooted in contemporary state-of-the-art knowledge in accessible ways that are immediately applicable to practice.

This book is about clinical practice with individuals. In no way does this suggest that working with clients one-on-one is the best modality. Individual, family, group, organizational, and community practice are all modalities central to the profession, and adequate practice requires recognition of the need for each (Mattaini, 1995). In day-to-day practice, however, many clients are seen individually, sometimes by design and sometimes because of situational realities.

Why do individual work? Is it not more important to work on community and policy levels, especially at moments in history in which the most vulnerable populations (social work's historic constituency) are facing increasing exploitation and oppression? This is a difficult issue, and some social work scholars have argued that community-level work is the only responsible choice and that the best way to help people is to build healthy communities (Specht, 1990; Specht & Courtney, 1994). Bertha Capon Reynolds (1934/1982) struggled with this question more than 60 years ago during the height of the Great Depression. Her resolution—and mine—was that the need for social action and advocacy is acute; at the same time, we cannot leave individuals to suffer unaided, and building healthier people also contributes to a healthier community. This is not an either/or choice.

AN ECOBEHAVIORAL APPROACH

Multiple practice "models" or approaches are available for social work practice. This book outlines one model, an *ecobehavioral* (see Lutzker, Frame, & Rice, 1982, for the origins of the term) approach. This model is highly collaborative and empowering and avoids pathologizing normal reactions to unfortunate circumstances and learning histories. Social workers can practice from this approach and call what they are doing "casework," "therapy," "treatment," "counseling," or "personal consultation." I personally prefer the last term because I believe it emphasizes the collaborative nature of the process and suggests similarities with other professional relationships (for example, in law, management, or finance) in which the professional outlines options, assists the client to understand the factors that are relevant, and guides and encourages the client to make effective decisions. I believe this model is closer to what social workers do, or should do, than is a medical model in which the worker "fixes" what is wrong with the client.

Because the approach presented here is firmly rooted in empirical data, practice based on this approach has a high likelihood of being effective. I include references to important examples and reviews of such work in the reference lists at the end of each chapter. Basing practice on demonstrably effective strategies is, of course, essential; each case, however, is in some ways unique, and many are unique. Practitioners often cannot simply select the "right" interventive protocol from a menu, as a physician might select a drug. Therefore, social workers also require a comprehensive and coherent conceptual framework to guide them in identifying the key factors operating in a particular case and in inventing new interventions when necessary. The present model is both based on empirical data and firmly grounded in comprehensive theory.

The ecobehavioral approach can often be effectively applied on a short-term basis. Contemporary practice, as in managed care, may place time limits on service. Behavioral approaches generally work relatively quickly, and time limits can be beneficial under certain circumstances. Professional practice encourages contracting with the client for brief blocks of sessions (sometimes several times) but requires that the extent of intervention ultimately be guided by the data—to work as quickly as possible, but no faster (see Gambrill, 1994, for a discussion of arbitrary time limits). Strictly arbitrary time limits may pose serious ethical problems.

I have been asked why I use the term *ecobehavioral*. Why not just *behavioral* (or the traditional social work term, *sociobehavioral*)? Although some practitioners from the behavioral social work community strongly disagree, I believe the ecosystems perspective (Meyer, 1995) and ecological models of practice (for example, Germain & Gitterman, 1996) have something important to teach us—that social workers may need to attend to not only the behavior of the individual but also the behavior of the multiple members of the multiple cultures (including family, organizational, neighborhood, ethnic, or even national cultures) within which the client is embedded. Using the term *culture* in this broad sense, it is often essential to work with the client to design family, organizational, peer, and other cultures that will support achieving the client's goals and maintenance of changes the client makes. Ultimately, social workers are not interested in simply changing behavior but in changing behavior–environment relations or more precisely in changing patterns of events embedded indivisibly in person and world (Lee, 1994). This model often involves linking the client to new cultures and modifying those that exist, for example, in the family or the peer group, to support positive change, and doing so requires a deeply contextualized perspective.

ORGANIZATION OF THIS BOOK

This book is organized as follows: Chapter 1 presents basic terms, principles, and theory that will be used throughout the book. Included is material that may be new even to readers with some familiarity with common behavioral principles; this material has emerged over the past decade or so and allows the approach to be applied in more complex areas of human and social functioning than in earlier treatments.

Chapter 2 covers engagement and assessment. Building an adequate relationship with the client is often essential both for gathering the data needed to complete an assessment and for motivating change. Effective practice also clearly requires adequate assessment. The area of assessment is one in which an ecobehavioral approach to clinical practice may provide particular advantages.

Chapters 3 through 5 outline general behavioral interventive strategies and techniques that are applicable across a broad range of clinical issues, including cognitive techniques. Chapter 6 is a brief, critical chapter outlining what is known about maintaining change once it has been achieved. Maintaining positive change has proved difficult for all practice approaches that have examined it. For example, in substance abuse treatment, the risk of relapse is high regardless of basic treatment approach, and similar issues often arise with regard to emotional, relationship, and many other human problems. Because of their propensity to actually collect data on client functioning, behaviorists were among the first to identify the problem clearly and have therefore focused significant energy on developing effective responses.

Chapters 7 through 10 focus on several common issues that social workers deal with in daily practice. The problems covered are depression and demoralization, relationship issues (particularly in the family), substance abuse, and severe mental and behavioral disorders (including what are commonly and, I argue, inaccurately labeled "personality disorders"). This selection of issues is not meant to suggest that these are the only problems clinical social workers see or that they are the most important; many forms of human pain can be equally devastating. I have chosen these particular issues because they are common among social work clients (including members of particularly vulnerable populations such as homeless and poor people and insular single-parent families), because they cover a broad range of concerns and therefore demonstrate the breadth of the approach, and because they are problems with which I have substantial clinical and programmatic experience.

INADEQUATE RESOURCES

Many social work clients experience severe problems with resource limitations, including extreme poverty, lack of adequate (or any) housing options, and lack of access to services (often associated with racism, sexism, homophobia, and other forms of oppression). Assisting clients to address these areas is an integral and organic part of clinical social work and one that may often be far more important than any "psychological" intervention. Assistance with these problems is often categorized separately as providing "concrete services" or working with "environmental problems." I do not make this artificial separation in this book.

These reality factors are often among the most critical variables involved in behavioral contingencies (behavior–environment relationships) in clinical situations and should therefore not be seen as a separate, and especially not as a separate and unequal, aspect of practice. In the chapters that follow, problems with inadequate tangible and social resources will therefore be integrated into the discussion. For example, poverty is often associated with depression and demoralization (as well as with each of the other clinical issues highlighted). The particular contribution of an ecobehavioral approach is surely not to notice poverty but rather to assist in understanding how poverty may contribute to demoralization and what potential options may therefore exist for ameliorating the effects.

CONCLUSION

In this brief introduction, I have sketched the reasons why I believe an ecobehavioral approach has much to offer contemporary social workers and their clients. There may be other approaches that are capable of doing an even better job (certainly improvements will come with time), but it is the responsibility of those who espouse these approaches to demonstrate their usefulness. In the meantime, I believe social workers have an ethical responsibility to familiarize themselves with an approach that substantial data suggest can make a profound difference in the lives of clients. A brief guide such as this one can only sketch the broadest outlines of the model, but perhaps this outline will provide motivation to look more closely at the details.

REFERENCES

Gambrill, E. (1994). What's in a name? Task-centered, empirical and behavioral practice. *Social Service Review, 68,* 578–599.

Gambrill, E. (in press). *Helping clients: A critical thinker's guide.* White Plains, NY: Longman.

Germain, C. B., & Gitterman, A. (1996). *The life model of social work practice* (2nd ed.). New York: Columbia University Press.

Granvold, D. K. (Ed.). (1994). *Cognitive and behavioral treatments: Methods and applications.* Pacific Grove, CA: Brooks/Cole.

Hayes, S. C. (1992). Verbal relations, time and suicide. In S. C. Hayes & L. J. Hayes (Eds.), *Understanding verbal relations* (pp. 109–118). Reno, NV: Context Press.

Kohlenberg, R. J., & Tsai, M. (1991). *Functional analytic psychotherapy: Creating intense and curative therapeutic relationships.* New York: Plenum Press.

Kohlenberg, R. J., & Tsai, M. (1994). Improving cognitive therapy for depression with functional analytic psychotherapy: Theory and case study. *Behavior Analyst, 17,* 305–319.

Lee, V. L. (1994). Organisms, things done, and the fragmentation of psychology. *Behavior and Philosophy, 22,* 7–48.

Lutzker, J. R., Frame, R. E., & Rice, J. M. (1982). Project 12-Ways: An ecobehavioral approach to the treatment and prevention of child abuse and neglect. *Education and Treatment of Children, 5,* 141–155.

Mattaini, M. A. (1995). Generalist practice: People and programs. In C. H. Meyer & M. A. Mattaini (Eds.), *The foundations of social work practice: A graduate text* (pp. 225–245). Washington, DC: NASW Press.

Meyer, C. H. (1993). *Assessment in social work practice.* New York: Columbia University Press.

Meyer, C. H. (1995). The ecosystems perspective: Implications for practice. In C. H. Meyer & M. A. Mattaini (Eds.), *The foundations of social work practice: A graduate text* (pp. 16–27). Washington, DC: NASW Press.

Reynolds, B. C. (1982). *Between client and community: A study in responsibility in social case work.* Washington, DC: National Association of Social Workers. (Original work published 1934)

Schwartz, A. (1983). Behavioral principles and approaches. In A. Rosenblatt & D. Waldfogel (Eds.), *Handbook of clinical social work* (pp. 202–228). San Francisco: Jossey-Bass.

Schwartz, A., & Goldiamond, I. (1975). *Social casework: A behavioral approach.* New York: Columbia University Press.

Specht, H. (1990). Social work and the popular psychotherapies. *Social Service Review, 64,* 345–357.

Specht, H., & Courtney, M. (1994). *Unfaithful angels: How social work has abandoned its mission.* New York: Free Press.

Thyer, B. A., Himle, J., & Santa, C. (1986). Applied behavior analysis in social and community action: A bibliography. *Behavior Analysis and Social Action, 5,* 14–16.

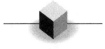

CHAPTER ONE

BASIC ECOBEHAVIORAL PRINCIPLES

Human behavior is embedded in a complex matrix of events and conditions to which it is responsive. The material in this chapter will introduce the principles of the science of behavior that explain how this occurs. This chapter introduces core behavioral principles, including recent (and perhaps at first glance, esoteric) concepts such as *rule-governance* and *equivalence relations*, with which contemporary social workers should be familiar. Although the principles are general to human behavior, the examples used are drawn from clinical practice to link the theory that underlies an ecobehavioral approach to its application by social workers.

Learning new practice approaches in-depth often involves learning a new language. For example, the precise meanings of *projective identification* or *defects of the self* (both used in contemporary psychodynamic practice) are not self-evident. The same is true for sophisticated understanding of ecobehavioral concepts. Because the terms used may be unfamiliar or the way they are used may be different than in everyday life, the risk of misunderstanding is substantial. For example, what people commonly call "negative reinforcement" is not reinforcement at all but punishment. (All reinforcement—positive or negative—by definition increases behavior; anything that decreases behavior is punishment.) Wherever possible I will define and use the standard terms, which often allow a level of precision and professional communication that is not otherwise possible.

CORE BEHAVIORAL PRINCIPLES

The defining tenet of behavioral theory is that human behavior is shaped by learning history—the relationships between one's actions and environmental events and conditions. The previous sentence as written is too simple, but it

1

does capture a central theoretical notion. More adequately, the science of behavior suggests that interactions of genetic and physiological factors, one's idiosyncratic life experiences, cultural patterns within which people have been embedded over the life course, and current conditions shape and maintain behavior.

The material that follows will clarify what is meant here by *behavior*, the multiple types of antecedents and consequences that affect it, and other concepts important to understanding complex human and social behavior. Most of the emphasis will be on *operant behavior* (roughly "voluntary" actions), because most clinical social work involves such behavior. A brief sketch of principles involved in *respondent behavior* (involuntary physical processes such as sweating) will be included for completeness.

What Is Behavior?

Contrary to popular (and often even professional!) misconceptions, contemporary behavioral theory applies to both public and private actions and includes motor, verbal, observational, and physiological–emotive events (Poppen, 1989). Clinically, acting or being violent, crying, listening to one's child, feeling tense, or thinking (in words or images) are all behavior, and crucially, all can be understood from the present theoretical framework. Cognitive–behavioral processes are therefore simply a subset of behavioral phenomena. For example, like other behavior, *self-talk* (such as saying to oneself, "this is intolerable") is shaped by life events. In fact, clients often "hear in their heads" (covert observational behavior) messages like "you'll never amount to anything"—rather like a tape (sometimes in the voice of a parent or other significant figure). Cognitive treatment can most simply be viewed as providing new learning experiences so that on some occasions, clients tell themselves, and hear, different messages.

Consequences

The core contribution of the science of behavior is that behavior is shaped by consequences. What "works" tends to be repeated; what does not work is not repeated. There are several important categories of consequences relevant to the development of clinical problems and to their resolution.

Positive Reinforcement. A positive reinforcer is defined as a consequence that leads to increased behavior in the future. It is roughly similar to a *reward*— a term that may be useful with clients, although technically one reinforces behavior and rewards people. The term *incentive* also is a useful rough

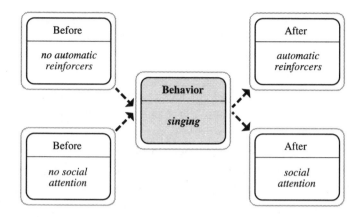

Figure 1-1. The positive reinforcement process.

synonym for a positive reinforcer. People act if effective incentives are in place. They may sing both because singing can be naturally reinforcing and for the attention they receive for it, for example. The process of positive reinforcement is shown in Figure 1-1.

Before the behavior, the person has fewer natural reinforcers and less attention. After the behavior, he or she has more of each. As another example, people sometimes take drugs (especially in the beginning) because of their physiological effects (they provide "automatic" reinforcement) and sometimes because of the social reinforcement received as part of a culture of drug-using peers.

Some reinforcers are biologically programmed, such as food, water, affection, and sensory and sexual stimulation. Others (*conditioned reinforcers*) are potentiated through association with primary or other learned reinforcers. Babies will not produce much behavior for money (unless it is shiny!), but many adults will. Some reinforcers may involve both genetic and learned processes—for example, most people like music, but tastes vary individually and culturally, based on experience.

The *schedules* on which reinforcers are delivered also are important. If a particular behavior "pays off" richly every time, a person may do it a lot (imagine a slot machine that gave an average of $5 for every two times you put in $1). Leaner schedules (in which behavior "pays off" less often) may produce less behavior, unless reinforcers are gradually faded from a richer schedule. There are many technically distinct schedules, but for clinical purposes, the most important concepts are the following:

- Rich schedules are often important to establish a behavior.
- Intermittent schedules (in which reinforcers follow behavior sometimes but not always) tend to produce robust patterns of behavior that often are maintained during reasonable periods of nonreinforcement.
- Gradually reducing the frequency, intensity, or amount of reinforcers delivered is often important for maintenance of change, so long as the reductions are not too extreme.

These principles have direct applicability in areas such as parenting, of course, but also apply in much more subtle ways. It is not uncommon in couples, for example, for one partner to reinforce richly in the beginning ("when courting"). Because such reinforcement involves effort, this pattern often gradually fades over time. In some cases (depending on many specifics of learning history) the other partner finds himself or herself working harder and harder to get what little reinforcement comes, leading to a situation of potential exploitation. In other cases, the couple "grows apart" as other environmental reinforcers become more important.

Because positive reinforcement has few negative side effects if properly handled and need not be done precisely to be effective (remember the power of intermittent schedules), it is the most important behavior change procedure in the entire human repertoire. It is a natural process that shapes everyone's behavior, and the closer clinical uses of reinforcement remain to *natural contingencies* (those occurring in the real world), the better. For example, if praise or smiles (which most everyone likes and responds to) work, it is better not to use artificial reinforcers such as food or money. When these natural reinforcers are not adequate (for example, to get people to get up early and go to work every day), more tangible incentives may be required (such as paychecks, although this situation is actually more complicated; people generally go to work to avoid losing a later paycheck, rather than to obtain immediate reinforcers). It is also possible to exploit people by using positive reinforcers if the schedule is too lean, for example, in some forms of "piece work."

Differential Reinforcement. One effective way to select which behaviors will occur more often and which less often is to reinforce some and not others. This is a crucial principle of effective parenting; paying attention when a child is "being good" instead of when he or she is acting up is a powerful intervention but one that is widely neglected in homes and schools. The same basic principle is also used, often intuitively, by effective social workers who notice and respond when clients take steps toward acting or thinking in new, potentially effective ways. Perhaps the most important variation is *differential reinforcement of incompatible behavior* (DRI), as in reinforcing children for doing schoolwork and not reinforcing for running around the room. Differential reinforcement is among the most powerful of behavioral tools, and many examples presented throughout this book rely on this principle. Another variation is differential reinforcement of other behavior (DRO), in which doing anything except the undesirable behavior is reinforced. This usually plays out as reinforcing increasing periods of time in which the behavior does not occur (and by definition, in which other behavior is happening, because so long as one is alive, one is behaving). Rates of behavior can also be reinforced (for example, differential reinforcement of low rates [DRL] or differential reinforcement of high rates [DRH]).

Shaping. Another powerful behavioral tool is *shaping*. In this process, reinforcement is provided for *successive approximations* gradually approaching the desired repertoire. A simple example is the way parents teach a young child to talk, first paying attention to practically any verbalization, but eventually differentially attending to those that sound like words (imitation also is involved in learning language). Many clients lack desired repertoires; for example, appropriate assertive and social behaviors. It is commonly useful to begin with simple first approximations, such as saying "good morning" to a woman at work, and then gradually work toward more difficult challenges such as asking someone at a party for a date. The social worker should ensure that valued reinforcers are available on rich enough schedules to shape and maintain such behavior.

Negative Reinforcement. *Negative reinforcement* may be the most misunderstood term in the entire behavioral lexicon. Negative reinforcement *increases* behavior that results in either escaping or avoiding an *aversive* (unpleasant) situation. The aversive event or condition is the *negative reinforcer*. Doing something unpleasant to people after they misbehave so they will not do it again, by definition, is not negative reinforcement; it is *punishment*. (Doing something unpleasant to people after they misbehave because it makes you feel better is retribution, which is not a behavioral strategy.) Remember, all reinforcement (positive or negative) by definition increases behavior.

Many behaviors that disturb clients have been shaped by negative reinforcement. People will do all kinds of surprising things to escape anxiety and other unpleasant emotional states, some of which they may not be aware of (Freud identified many of these defense mechanisms), ranging from forgetting to displacing emotions onto others to repeating actions over and over in a compulsive way. Figure 1-2 depicts an example of negative reinforcement. Aggressive children often learn that, if they act aggressively or coercively, they can escape unpleasant demands, which in turn can lead to escalation of coercive exchanges in the family—see chapter 8 for further discussion.

Nonreinforcement. Behavior that does not produce reinforcers becomes less likely in the future. This apparently simple principle provides a potentially powerful interventive tool. Because eliminating the reinforcer can reduce behavior, planned nonreinforcement is often an effective way to reduce the rate of undesirable behavior. The planned nonreinforcement process is outlined in Figure 1-3. (The rather unfortunate technical term for this process is *extinction.*) One major challenge with planned nonreinforcement is to ensure that the reinforcer is always withheld; otherwise, what is being set up is an intermittent schedule of reinforcement, and the behavior may then become strongly resistant to change. For example, if a teacher usually ignores minor disruptive behavior, but sometimes attends to it (or if peers do), the disruptions may become difficult to eliminate.

Punishment. Technically, punishment involves changing consequences to reduce the rate of a behavior. One familiar approach is to present an aversive event or condition after the undesirable behavior (for example, spanking or yelling); another is to remove a reinforcer (for example, levying a fine—taking away a positive). This second approach is often called *response cost.* Punishment is a controversial procedure among behavioral social workers. Most agree with

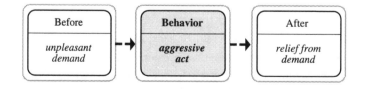

Figure 1-2. The negative reinforcement (escape) process.

Clinical Practice with Individuals

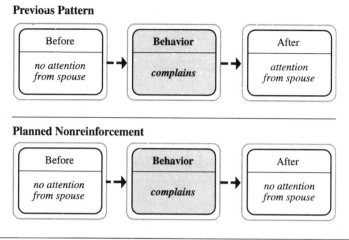

Previous Pattern

Before	Behavior	After
no attention from spouse	*complains*	*attention from spouse*

Planned Nonreinforcement

Before	Behavior	After
no attention from spouse	*complains*	*no attention from spouse*

Figure 1-3. The planned nonreinforcement (extinction) process.

Skinner (1953) that positive reinforcement procedures for building alternatives are usually more effective. Several issues with punishment exist:

- As long as the reinforcer that maintains the behavior remains available, the person still is "inclined" to display the behavior. For example, an employee whose pay is docked for being late to work may still prefer to sleep in if no one monitors attendance. As a result, it may be necessary to monitor closely when punishing.
- Punishment teaches the use of coercion. Children who experience high levels of punishment while growing up tend to act coercively toward the punisher when the opportunity presents itself and later in life with their own children, spouses, employees, or others.
- In some cases, people adapt to modest levels of punishment, and it may become necessary to use increasingly harsh punishments to maintain the reduction in behavior.

All of these issues suggest that punishment is often a poor first choice for changing behavior.

Some forms of punishment may be less problematic; small self-imposed fines that are easy to avoid, for example, can be useful in self-management programs. Figure 1-4 shows this simple and effective strategy. A client seen in a medical setting may need to follow certain dietary restrictions. An arrangement can be established in which he pays a $1 fine to his secretary each time he eats an undesirable lunch (for example, a cheeseburger and french fries) instead of salad

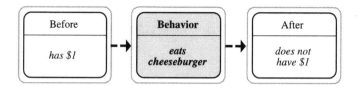

Figure 1-4. A mild punishment strategy useful for self-management.

and bread as listed in his diet. A simple program such as this, so long as it is regularly monitored and embedded in a system of social reinforcers from the social worker and secretary, can be surprisingly powerful (see chapter 5 for more details about self-management). In life-threatening or dangerous circumstances, the use of punishment in conjunction with reinforcement for alternatives may occasionally be justified (see, for example, Sajwaj, Libet, & Agras, 1974). There is significant risk, however, that if coercive punishment works (is reinforced) in one situation, it may be used in other situations. Punishment may come to be relied on when it is not required, resulting in an increasingly coercive social environment.

One hybrid procedure that is sometimes viewed as an example of extinction but that is perhaps more accurately viewed as a mild form of response cost is *time-out*, a procedure useful in parenting if used in conjunction with reinforcement procedures for alternatives. If a child misbehaves, under some circumstances he or she can be briefly placed in a location that offers few reinforcers for a brief time (no more than one minute per year of age); as a result, the rate of the problem behavior will often decline. The specifics of the procedure can be found in standard behavioral parent education books (for example, Patterson, 1975; Sloane, 1976/1988).

For these reasons, clinicians should always rely on the least coercive strategy consistent with client and family well-being. Because punishment can damage relationships and lead to aggression or depression, it is a risky procedure that should be used only in emergencies or when nothing else will work. Many alternative procedures are available and are discussed in subsequent chapters.

Antecedents

Behavior is selected by its consequences—the rate at which a behavior occurs changes based on consequences for similar actions in the past. Events and conditions (including environmental factors and private experiences—those known

Clinical Practice with Individuals

only to the person) that precede a behavior (antecedents) also influence its rate, largely because of their connections with consequences. There are three classes of antecedents that are particularly important in clinical work: (1) occasions when particular consequences are likely, (2) motivating antecedents that affect sensitivity to consequences, and (3) structural factors that make the behavior possible. In addition, two specialized types of antecedents (special cases of one or more of the three already listed) exist: modeling and rules. Each of these will be introduced in the following paragraphs.

Occasions. An occasion (a discriminative stimulus or S^D) is an event or condition that "signals" that reinforcement for a behavior is available. A client may learn, for example, that certain forms of assertive behavior will produce a positive result with friends, whereas with her abusive partner the outcome of the behavior might be different. Human behavior often comes under the stimulus control (the process in which the connection between the occasion and the consequence of the behavior is made) of highly complex combinations of circumstances. For example, in conditional discrimination, an occasion (such as a child's request to play) may prompt a particular behavior (the parent playing with the child) in the presence of one person (e.g., a social worker providing parent training) but not if that person is not present. Questions of stimulus control must often be carefully considered in constructing new repertoires and in planning for their maintenance.

Motivating Antecedents. Some antecedent conditions or events affect the level of a person's motivation to act. In recent years, behavior analysts have learned a good deal about how this works. Changing environmental and physiological conditions can increase or decrease sensitivity to particular consequences. For example, a person who experiences a sudden decrease in positive exchanges at home may come to value friends at work more highly and may spend more time with them.[1]

For example, a client whose husband of 20 years had recently left her found that the reinforcers offered by friends became more important to her; as a result, she contacted and spent time with friends more often. (This was a healthy

---

[1]Those events that increase sensitivity are technically called establishing operations (EOs); those events that decrease sensitivity are called abolishing operations. Both are referred to in this book as motivating variables, but in the behavioral community the term EO (pronounced "eee-oh") is commonly used. Motivating variables (establishing operations) both affect sensitivity to consequences and evoke behavior that will produce the consequences (Michael, 1993).

response and followed a predictable period of sadness and withdrawal resulting from the loss of valued reinforcers.) The way the process appeared to work is shown in Figure 1-5. Living alone (the motivating antecedent) resulted in a lack of social reinforcers. The client therefore became more sensitive to such reinforcers, and as a result behavior producing social contact increased.

Deprivation (of many kinds) is among the most powerful of motivating antecedents. People with few resources (physical or social) often live in a state of generalized deprivation and are often highly sensitized to whatever reinforcers may be available—for example, those offered by addictive drugs. Satiation, in contrast, decreases sensitivity (people usually only eat so much of even the most delicious food). Exposure to novel reinforcers ("try it, you'll like it") often establishes sensitivity to those reinforcers. This process, called *reinforcer sampling*, can be useful, for example, with low-income youths who commonly have not experienced a wide range of life experiences that they might find highly reinforcing but are not potentiated until the person is exposed to them. Verbal (from others or oneself) and observational behaviors also can increase sensitivity—advertising is built on these strategies.

Structural Factors. Social workers commonly recognize that there are environmental and personal limitations in cases that affect the possibility of some behaviors on the part of a client, collateral, or other person. These structural factors may make it possible or impossible, easy or difficult, for the person to act in particular ways. For example, if a client on welfare does not have child care or transportation available, it may not be possible for her to take a job, even if everyone involved thinks that would be best. People themselves have limitations, as well; for example, some children with fetal alcohol syndrome lack the capacity to learn rapidly enough to succeed in regular schools.

Structural factors must always be considered in planning with clients. In some cases, the client and worker may set an objective of employment, because it is a

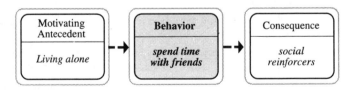

Figure 1-5. A motivating condition increases sensitivity to a reinforcer and evokes behavior that produces the reinforcer.

Clinical Practice with Individuals

step toward the client's basic goals: gaining access to highly valued reinforcers and thinking about himself or herself in more positive ways (see the discussion of self-talk later in this chapter). If, however, resources needed to achieve that goal, such as transportation or child care, are not available, the clinician and client may need to think about other ways to achieve the basic goals.

Imitation. Luckily, people do not need to try everything themselves to find out what "works" in life. Sometimes they can learn from what they are told by others (see the section "Rule-Governed Behavior" later in this chapter), but often the most effective learning comes from seeing how other people do things. A person who observes how his or her parents respond to things their children do will often find himself or herself doing the same when he or she becomes a parent. If a person watches someone else model an action that results in reinforcement, that person is likely to imitate the behavior. (Skinner, 1987, p. 68), suggests that imitation may have genetic roots.) The "social learning" approach to understanding human behavior places particular emphasis on how a person learns to imitate what is modeled by others (Bandura, 1986).

Imitation is not only involved in the development of many clinical problems, it also provides a valuable strategy for teaching clients new and potentially more effective behaviors. This strategy commonly involves modeling alternatives, providing opportunities to imitate (rehearse), and then gradually shaping more and more adequate repertoires. Modeling and rehearsal are effective techniques for use in groups (for example, when teaching assertive skills or alternatives to violence) and also are highly applicable to work with individuals. Many kinds of behavior can be taught through imitation, including how people describe themselves and the world.

Private Experiences

Many behaviors are only directly observable by the person displaying those behaviors, although other people may be able to infer these behaviors from what they can see. Examples of such behaviors include sensations (for example, pain), observation (noticing something in the environment through the senses, or imagining similar events), and self-talk (what one says to oneself). Many of these private experiences are important for clinical work. Cognitive therapists have concentrated extensively in this area, especially on self-talk, and many of the interventions they have developed are presented in subsequent chapters.

Private experiences are also behavior and can be shaped and maintained by antecedents and consequences in the same ways that overt behaviors are. For example, people often verbally describe contingencies (these descriptions are technically called *rules*) to themselves—self-talk—or to others. These verbal descriptions are shaped by imitation and reinforcement from others and through personal experience, all of which may lead to biased or inaccurate descriptions. If a client says, "There is no escape from this situation," he or she is unlikely to take any sort of action; one component of empowerment involves changes in such self-talk.

Some cognitive–behavioral theorists—Albert Ellis, for example—view self-talk in a way that is largely consistent with the way it is being presented here. (There are, however, differences in relative attributions of causality. Behaviorists tend to emphasize the ultimate importance of environmental factors, whereas rational emotive behavior therapists such as Ellis see the individual as an autonomous initiator to a greater extent.) Others, such as Aaron Beck, believe that hypothesized (but unfortunately ultimately untestable) cognitive "structures," such as schemas, also are required for a full explanation (Beck, Freeman, & Associates, 1990). As discussed in chapter 4, although these issues are often important for the development of new interventions, they often are far less important in day-to-day practice. Within an ecobehavioral approach, the simplest model that can account for the facts is preferred (Occam's Razor, the scientific principle of parsimony). For this reason, what one says to oneself as listener is seen here in ways similar to what one says to someone else.

Emotions. Although "methodological behaviorists" early in the 20th century avoided discussing emotions, feelings are among the areas that modern behaviorists and clinical social workers deal with most frequently in work with clients. Emotions are basically states of the body (visceral behaviors) that are associated with other events. Situations in which one has previously been punished, for example, are likely to make one feel "anxious," whereas the loss of important sources of reinforcers is likely to make one feel sad or, under certain conditions, depressed. From a behavioral perspective, emotions experienced are never seen as abnormal but rather as natural responses to current conditions and life history. As such, emotions are ordinarily amenable to change, given different experiences. In some cases, emotions (in particular, some forms of mood and psychotic disorders) appear to be so deeply grounded in biology that pharmacological interventions may be necessary. Other forms of behavior are commonly associated with emotions in predictable ways—what one says to oneself (self-talk), for example, can deepen or attenuate emotional arousal. Clients may become anxious, for example, when in the presence of aspects of the environment associated with previous aversive experiences. (This behavior is known as *respondent conditioning*, discussed later in this chapter.) All of these issues will be discussed in detail later in this book.

Rule-Governed Behavior. A basic behavioral principle with considerable empirical support is that consequences should follow behavior closely to influence its rate. Effective human beings, however, need to learn how to "defer gratification" and how to work toward distant goals. People also commonly act because someone else tells them what the consequences will be, even though the actor has never performed the behavior and experienced the consequences before. Behaviors of these types are not under the control of immediate, direct-acting contingencies, but rather are called *rule-governed* behaviors. Although many complexities are involved, basically a *rule* is a verbal description of a contingency (for example, "When my boss is in a good mood, if I ask nicely, I am likely to get what I want"). Rules as stated are often fragmentary and may leave out the occasion ("when my boss is in a good mood") or the consequence and may simply be stated as advice ("ask nicely"), but the missing pieces are implied. Rules are often stated privately as self-talk; for example, many clients have learned rules such as, "No matter what I do, no one will like me." Such rules are addressed directly by cognitive intervention.

Many important rules are hard to follow. For example, many students find it difficult to study consistently throughout a term if they are evaluated only by a final examination; they procrastinate, and some clients do so beyond the point of no return. One dimension of the problem is that the consequence is delayed; perhaps more central is that there are, at any moment, many other competing reinforcers, and whether one studies at this moment will have only a tiny effect on the final outcome. Situations that involve small, cumulative effects can be difficult for everyone and require well-established rule-governed repertoires. Many clients have not had the consistent experiences needed to shape such rule governance. For example, violent youths commonly act in response to direct-acting contingencies, lacking the rule-governed repertoires that could result in better-quality, but delayed, reinforcers (Mattaini, Twyman, Chin, & Nam, 1996).

Self-management techniques (chapter 5) can be of substantial use in such situations. Malott, Whaley, and Malott (1993) suggested that what is actually occurring in rule governance is that the person acts to escape from an immediate covert aversive. For example, when told that, if you mail in a coupon today, you will receive a check for $500 in two weeks, you are likely to do so, even though the consequence is delayed. According to Malott et al., you experience the possible loss of the $500 as a current aversive until you act to avoid it.

Equivalence Relations. Although there is no necessary connection among them, you learned at some point that "3," "three," and "III" mean the same thing and are (under some circumstances) equivalent. Technically, 3, three, and III participate in an *equivalence relation:* $3 \approx$ three $\approx$ III. Note that members of an equivalence relation need not be the same in all ways, only that they are functionally equivalent in some way. Equivalence relations can include antecedents (for example, behavior in one classroom may come to resemble that in another), the behaviors themselves, and the consequences (Sidman, 1994; see also Hayes, 1991, for a related approach). Note that an equivalence relation is not really a "thing"—rather multiple different words, events, people, and so forth evoke the same results. Racial and gender prejudices, for example, are rooted in overgeneralized and inaccurate equivalences.

Equivalence relations are among the most exciting areas of current basic behavioral research. Although they may appear complicated, they have substantial clinical importance, and the concepts are more accessible than they may seem. Hayes (1992) and others (for example, Dougher & Hackbert, 1994) suggested that depressed clients often demonstrate verbal equivalence relations such as

$$\text{me} \approx \text{failure} \approx \text{worthless.}$$

As a result, situations that evoke "me" also may evoke "failure" and so forth. If a client has formed such relations and also learned rules such as, "No matter what I do, people don't like me," it is easy to see how he or she can become locked in a downward emotional spiral. Equivalence may be one factor in suicide in which the client has formed equivalences between "myself" and "terrible situation" (this argument roughly follows Hayes, 1992). Under those circumstances, the client may come to believe that to escape from the situation he or she must escape from himself or herself as well. Working clinically with clients to achieve changes in equivalence relations (see chapter 4) is a particularly exciting area of emerging work.

Clinical Practice with Individuals

The Self. A related area that has received attention recently by behaviorists is the formation of the "self." The self will be discussed in detail in chapter 10, but a few comments may be useful here. Rather than viewing the self as a cognitive structure, ecobehavioral clinicians view experiencing a coherent self as learned behavior based on the same principles as other behavior (Kohlenberg & Tsai, 1991). This concept is important because it is hopeful; for example, rather than viewing a person as having a "personality disorder" that is seen as "a disorder of the entire person" (Davis & Millon, 1994), an ecobehavioral social worker views the issue as overlearned patterns of private and public behaviors (Mattaini, 1994). Seen in that way, there is no theoretical reason why alternative patterns cannot be learned.

Respondent Behavior

Ecobehavioral practice emphasizes operant or "voluntary" behavior because this is where most client difficulties usually lie. There are times, however, when respondent conditioning is relevant. For example, in phobias, previously neutral environmental conditions or events come to elicit anxiety through being paired with aversive events. For example, a client experienced panic attacks when he returned to an area where a bomb had gone off on a previous visit. The street scene (conditioned stimulus) produced anxiety (the response) by being paired with the explosion (the unconditioned stimulus). How a neutral event begins to elicit anxiety often is not as clear-cut as in this example, particularly when it occurs in early life. Ordinarily, it is not necessary with panic attacks, phobias, or other anxiety-related difficulties to locate the origin of the problem (which of course could not be changed anyway). The primary interventive strategy in such circumstances is to work with clients to expose themselves to the anxiety-provoking situation repeatedly without external negative effects (exposure), as a result of which the strength of the conditioned response fades. Although this is the basic paradigm, there are many crucial details required for effective intervention; these will be discussed in later chapters.

CONTINGENCIES

This chapter defines and provides examples of behavior, consequences, and antecedents. The relationships among these are called *contingencies*. Specifically, the relationship between a behavior and its consequence, the central core of behavioral theory, is a *two-term contingency*. Notice that the crucial relationship is behavior–consequence, not stimulus–response (which applies only to the narrower class of respondent behavior discussed previously). With the addition of the occasion, we have a three-term contingency (for example, when homework is completed, the adolescent asks to use the car, and he or she is given permission). In clinical social work, however, context also often matters; the previous example may be true on some days of the week and not on others. As a result, the contingencies of interest may be four-term or even more complex. In many situations, there are competing and concurrent contingencies in place, which of course makes analysis difficult. People generally operate in "a sea of contingencies" (Malott, Whaley, & Malott, 1993, p. 378).

There are some ways to make sense of all of this, however. The matching law[2] provides substantial clinical guidance here (McDowell, 1988). Roughly, the matching law says that the relative rate of a behavior depends on the relative availability of reinforcers for that behavior compared with all other available reinforcers.

In applied situations, the matching law has several practical implications. To increase the rate of a behavior, you can increase reinforcement for that action while holding constant other reinforcers or decrease the availability of other sources of reinforcement. To decrease behavior, you can reduce reinforcers for that behavior *or* increase availability of other reinforcers (either contingent on alternative behaviors or simply free, noncontingent reinforcers). For example, antisocial behavior often can be substantially reduced by providing rich alternative sources of reinforcement, without even directly addressing the undesirable behavior. The matching law, which accounts for more than 90 percent of the variance in behavior in every study reported, has important implications for clinical work as well as for programming and policy making (see, for example, Epling & Pierce, 1983; Mattaini, 1991; McDowell, 1988; Vuchinich & Tucker, 1988).

---

[2]The form of the matching law that accounts for the rate of a single behavior in a particular environmental context is given in the following equation:

$$B = \frac{kr}{r + r_e} \, ,$$

where B is the rate of behavior, k is the (asymptotic) maximum rate of behavior, r is the rate of reinforcement available for the behavior, and r_e is the rate of "extraneous" reinforcement available in the contextual situation. Of course, not all reinforcers can be substituted for others—water cannot take the place of food, for example. In general, however, the more reinforcement of other kinds available in a particular situation (r_e), the lower the relative frequency of the behavior of interest (see McDowell, 1988, for further detail).

From an ecobehavioral perspective, the actions of the client, the social worker, family members, and representatives of the many systems that have positive or negative effects on clients are influenced by the contingencies within which their behavior is embedded. Analysis of available incentives and punishments (including often subtle social consequences conditioned through long experience) is crucial for effective clinical work. Intervention always involves affecting the contingencies of some behavior on the part of some people. This intervention may be as simple as the social worker providing new rules and encouragement in the clinical session or as complicated as working with clients to restructure the culture of their families and the other networks within which those in turn are embedded.

ECOBEHAVIORAL PRACTICE

The model of practice presented here is firmly rooted both in the ecosystems perspective indigenous to and almost universally accepted in contemporary social work and in the science of behavior (including behavior analysis and cultural analysis and design). The two have much to offer each other, but commonly they have not been adequately synthesized. This lack of synthesis has caused several problems. Excessive attention has sometimes been paid to client behavior rather than that of others in the client's life-space, because the client is more easily accessible. Lack of familiarity with the state-of-the-art in the science of behavior often leaves ecosystemic clinicians and clients to fend for themselves without the use of the most effective available tools for addressing the issues they identify. Finally, an emphasis on changing behavior without designing environmental supports to maintain the change, not surprisingly, often results in only short-lived success.

The ecobehavioral model, in addition to being grounded in current theoretical and empirical advances, encourages the social worker to view human action in context. The goal of clinical work most often involves exposing the client to new networks of social contingencies (new *cultures* in behavioral terms) or encouraging different practices in those with which the client is already involved. These cultures, including those of families, friendship networks, organizations, or communities of many kinds, are the most likely sources of ongoing support for changes desired by clients.

In clinical practice with individuals, intervention at these larger levels is often indirect. The practitioner may and often should have contact with collaterals involved in systems that have or could have an impact on the client. However, often the worker and client spend much of their consultation time identifying ways the client can take the steps required, for example, to join a different organization, to change the microculture of his or her family, or even to construct a new network to provide him or her with social support. Although the social worker is often a critical source of contingencies supporting change in the early stages, he or she should think constantly about how to work toward the point at which natural contingencies can take over.

The Problem of Coercive Environments

Many clients live in coercive circumstances—environments in which threats and punishment are common and severe. Coercion produces many negative side effects, including depression, aggression, and hopelessness (Sidman, 1989). Coercion (often subtle) can ruin the relationship between a couple, lead to the development of an escalating spiral of aggression between child and parent, or destroy morale in an organization or a sense of community in a neighborhood. Unfortunately, coercion often works—in the short run. For example, beating a child may lead to a reduction in undesirable behavior. However, in many circumstances, the problem behavior is likely to return, although it may become more covert; in all circumstances the use of coercion teaches both parties involved that coercion is an appropriate and effective way of getting what one wants.

American society has refined coercion to a fine art, and the results are clear: the rate of people incarcerated has increased threefold (without a significant drop in crime), nearly 50 percent of marriages end in divorce, and 25,000 homicides occur every year. Those who are poor or otherwise vulnerable experience far more coercive circumstances than people who are privileged. Many social work clients are members of the former groups, and an important interventive goal is often to reduce exposure to aversive conditions and events and increase access to more reinforcing environments.

The Behavioral Ecomap as Key Metaphor

The behavioral ecomap is a graphic depiction of the contingency network within which a client is embedded. Social workers have made extensive use of such graphic tools, which enable the worker and the client to examine the client's situation in an organic way (Hartman, 1995; Mattaini, 1993). Detailed behavioral ecomaps and other graphic tools are particularly valuable at later stages of the assessment and are discussed in the next chapter. A simple image such as that shown in Figure 1-6, however, is a key metaphor for ecobehavioral practice.

A core notion in ecobehavioral practice is that most clients are experiencing events or conditions that are too aversive and often too few that are reinforcing. Such exchanges with environmental systems are often, but not always, reciprocal and may be contingent (responsive to the individual's behavior) or noncontingent (not related to that behavior).

Both the specifics present (such as the abusive treatment the client in Figure 1-6 receives from her boyfriend) and the overall configuration (the client in Figure 1-6 receives little social reinforcement from anywhere) are relevant to understanding the client's situation and may be important focal issues to be addressed in clinical work. Although such a broad view is not always required, in the majority of social work cases, some attention to the overall case situation may be important. This perspective is useful for understanding the issues present contextually and also may help in identifying potentially useful, but untapped, resources.

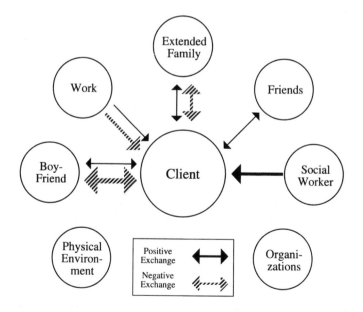

Figure 1-6. A simple ecomap depicting the ecobehavioral situation of a young woman with serious depression. Width of arrows indicates strength of transactions.

Ecobehavioral Practice Is Hopeful

Perhaps the most crucial point to be made about ecobehavioral practice is that it offers a hopeful perspective. If behavior is shaped and maintained by experience, problems can in theory be solved by helping the client to access new experiences. There are limits, of course, because there is much we do not yet know and the resources required are not always available. Still, beginning with the assumption that the causes of most human problems lie in webs of contingency interlocks that may be amenable to intervention by client and worker (rather than in intrapersonal pathology) suggests that change may usually be possible.

The core of clinical social work practice is intervention to change the adaptive fit between person and environment. Although many cases have much in common (for example, physiological dependence in addiction), every case also is unique. For this reason, the social worker and client ordinarily should engage in a process of individualizing assessment before beginning intervention. At the same time, the social worker should forge an effective relationship with the client, not one based only on offering social reinforcers to the client—who may not experience many of those—but one that profoundly helps the client in the long-term. Chapter 2 covers approaches for engaging the client and conducting a thorough assessment.

REFERENCES

Bandura, A. (1986). *Social foundations of thought and action: A social-cognitive theory.* Englewood Cliffs, NJ: Prentice Hall.

Beck, A. T., Freeman, A., & Associates. (1990). *Cognitive therapy of personality disorders.* New York: Guilford Press.

Davis, R. D., & Millon, T. (1994). Can personalities be disordered? Yes! In S. A. Kirk & S. D. Einbinder (Eds.), *Controversial issues in mental health* (pp. 40–47). Boston: Allyn & Bacon.

Dougher, M. J., & Hackbert, L. (1994). A behavior-analytic account of depression and a case report using acceptance-based procedures. *Behavior Analyst, 17,* 321–334.

Epling, W. F., & Pierce, W. D. (1983). Applied behavior analysis: New directions from the laboratory. *Behavior Analyst, 6,* 27–37.

Hartman, A. (1995). Diagrammatic assessment of family relationships. *Families in Society, 76,* 111–122.

Hayes, S. C. (1991). A relational control theory of stimulus equivalence. In L. J. Hayes & P. N. Chase (Eds.), *Dialogues on verbal behavior* (pp. 19–44). Reno, NV: Context Press.

Hayes, S. C. (1992). Verbal relations, time and suicide. In S. C. Hayes & L. J. Hayes (Eds.), *Understanding verbal relations* (pp. 109–118). Reno, NV: Context Press.

Kohlenberg, R. J., & Tsai, M. (1991). *Functional analytic psychotherapy: Creating intense and curative therapeutic relationships.* New York: Plenum Press.

Malott, R. W., Whaley, D. L., & Malott, M. E. (1993). *Elementary principles of behavior* (2nd ed.). Englewood Cliffs, NJ: Prentice Hall.

Mattaini, M. A. (1991). Choosing weapons for the war on "crack": An operant analysis. *Research on Social Work Practice, 1,* 188–213.

Mattaini, M. A. (1993). *More than a thousand words: Graphics for clinical practice.* Washington, DC: NASW Press.

Mattaini, M. A. (1994). Can personalities be disordered? No! In S. A. Kirk & S. Einbinder (Eds.), *Controversial issues in mental health* (pp. 48–56). Boston: Allyn & Bacon.

Mattaini, M. A., Twyman, J. S., Chin, W., & Nam, K. (1996). Youth violence. In M. A. Mattaini & B. A. Thyer (Eds.), *Finding solutions to social problems: Behavioral strategies for change.* Washington, DC: APA Books.

McDowell, J. J. (1988). Matching theory in natural human environments. *Behavior Analyst, 11,* 95–109.

Michael, J. L. (1993). *Concepts and principles of behavior analysis.* Kalamazoo, MI: Society for the Advancement of Behavior Analysis.

Patterson, G. R. (1975). *Families: Applications of social learning to family life.* Champaign, IL: Research Press.

Poppen, R. L. (1989). Some clinical implications of rule-governed behavior. In S. C. Hayes (Ed.), *Rule-governed behavior: Cognition, contingencies, and instructional control* (pp. 325–357). New York: Plenum Press.

Sajwaj, T., Libet, J., & Agras, S. (1974). Lemon juice therapy: The control of life-threatening rumination in a six-month-old infant. *Journal of Applied Behavior Analysis, 7,* 557–563.

Sidman, M. (1989). *Coercion and its fallout.* Boston: Authors Cooperative.

Sidman, M. (1994). *Equivalence relations and behavior: A research story.* Boston: Authors Cooperative.

Skinner, B. F. (1953). *Science and human behavior.* New York: Free Press.

Skinner, B. F. (1987). *Upon further reflection.* Englewood Cliffs, NJ: Prentice Hall.

Sloane, H. N. (1988). *The good kid book.* Champaign, IL: Research Press. (Original work published 1976)

Vuchinich, R. E., & Tucker, J. A. (1988). Contributions from behavioral theories of choice to an analysis of alcohol abuse. *Journal of Abnormal Psychology, 97,* 181–195.

CHAPTER TWO

ASSESSMENT

Although knowing how to intervene is the final test, the core of professional practice is the assessment. Only by completing an adequate assessment can the social worker–client team decide how to intervene and with
what. Because every case is different, simply identifying a categorical problem
(such as "depression" or "parenting problem") is not sufficient to make a plan
responsive to the unique qualities of the case. Assessment commonly is itera-
tive, producing hypotheses that are tested and refined in the consulting room
and the client's life-space. The results produce new data that can be fed back
into the assessment process. This chapter provides an outline of the essential
steps involved in completing an adequate ecobehavioral assessment.

The primary emphasis in this chapter is on assessment strategies that can
be implemented relatively rapidly, given the tremendous time pressures present
in contemporary practice. Although assessment can often be done quickly, it
cannot leave out any essential steps and still be regarded as professional. The
social worker cannot send every depressed client for medication without exploring possible sources of the problem in the client's life or send everyone
with an alcohol problem to a 12-step program. Performing assessments quickly
is a requirement dictated by reality; taking the time necessary to do so is an
ethical imperative.

In most cases, to complete an adequate assessment and intervene effectively, clinical social workers should achieve respectful and empathic working relationships with clients. Establishing a relationship in which both
worker and client have authentic voices (Lowery & Mattaini, 1996) is not
sufficient for change in any but the most exceptional cases, but in most
cases it is necessary. Before looking at the stages of assessment, therefore, a
few reflections on engaging clients and on building trusting consultative
relationships may be useful.

ENGAGING THE CLIENT

A social worker must build a positive, collaborative relationship with a client to be helpful. Workers who authentically communicate empathy and respect to clients probably have the best outcomes, and the importance of mutual, collaborative relationships between worker and client has long been recognized in social work (Coady, 1993). The professional relationship is not an end in itself; for example, if a client's major problem is social isolation, the ultimate purpose of professional consultation should be to help the client build relationships in the natural environment, not for the social worker to become a paid friend. Although social workers get a lot back from work with clients, the clinical relationship exists for the client. In an important sense, it is a one-way street.

In behavioral terms, the components of an effective professional relationship are relatively straightforward. Clients often have a story to tell but lack the opportunity or skills to do so. Clients' descriptions of environmental events and conditions and their own reactions to them are shaped and potentially biased by earlier life experiences, but such events still constitute important data. The effective social worker acts as a nonpunitive audience who lets the client describe these things in his or her own way and who can then work with him or her to identify the most important factors in the case. In traditional psychoanalysis, the nonpunitive audience provided by the therapist allows previously punished material to gradually emerge. (According to Skinner, because this material does not produce punishment, but is also not reinforced, those previously punished behaviors weaken and fade. Refer to page 10 of Skinner, 1989.)

Many clients have experienced substantial punishment from others around them for honestly experiencing or discussing their experiences, and as a result, these clients may have difficulty finding their "voices." For example, many battered women are afraid to discuss what is happening with the battering partner and may also fear talking about it with family or friends. The experience of having someone listen and reinforce telling one's story can have profound effects. Previous life experience often has taught clients that honesty will be punished; when the social worker does not punish, the client will often come to share increasingly personal material. An empathic worker also communicates that he or she hears and, to some extent, shares the client's experiences, including emotions (a process rooted in imitation; see Skinner, 1989). Once trust is established, the worker also can help the client to clarify experiences and situations that have not yet been put into words. Some degree of worker self-disclosure can help, as long as it is guided by the client's needs rather than the worker's inclination. In addition, nonpunitive listening communicates respect and may thereby help the client to construct equivalences such as

$$me \approx valuable \approx worth\ taking\ time.$$

Being heard is a valued source of reinforcement; respectful social behaviors that suggest that the social worker sees the client as an equal, rather than a member of a devalued class, are almost universally valued.

Being nonpunitive, empathic, and respectful is an important beginning; however, other crucial dimensions of an effective consulting relationship exist as well. If the social worker is not to rely on coercion but is expected to do something to produce a change (in someone's behavior), the remaining option is to use positive reinforcement to construct and strengthen effective client repertoires and actions by others that will benefit the client. The worker often must become a source of valued reinforcers (usually social) for the client. At later stages, when the client must take difficult steps, the worker can then function as a "bridge"—a principal source of reinforcement for those steps until natural contingencies take over. In addition, the worker usually also wants to become a trusted source of effective rules about the connections between client actions and probable consequences, because he or she will often encourage the client to undertake new and perhaps anxiety-provoking tasks.

In most cases, the worker's first challenge is to induce the client to return (or in less voluntary circumstances to work with the clinician in an honest way). If the session provides valued reinforcers (which may range from empathic understanding to simple agreement, or from immediate symptom relief to a feeling of hope), this becomes more likely. What is valued varies from person to person, although some things are likely to be useful in many cases. For example, recognition of positive aspects of what the client says or does has a double advantage: it may reinforce doing or saying more of those things (supporting client strengths) while establishing the worker as a source of reinforcers. Positive statements about the client's behavior also may come to participate in equivalence relations such as

$$my\ behavior \approx effective \approx successful.$$

How the social worker becomes a trusted source of rules also will be idiosyncratic to a particular worker–client configuration. Sue and Zane (1987) suggested that credibility is particularly crucial in cross-cultural work.

Clinical Practice with Individuals

Although credibility is more difficult to achieve in cross-cultural situations, it is challenging in most clinical work. Some general principles that may be of help are:

+ If the worker resembles people whose advice and view of the world the client has come to trust, he or she starts with an advantage.
+ If the worker describes situations in the client's life in terms congruent with the client's experience, credibility may increase.
+ If the client finds that predictions the worker makes prove to be true, he or she may come increasingly to trust the worker's perceptions of connections between behavior and consequences—the worker becomes a trusted source of rules.

Figure 2-1 shows examples of worker statements that may encourage the client to share and that can deepen the professional relationship. This deepening may then result in a more accurate and adequate assessment in addition to potentiating the worker as a valued source of reinforcers and rules during intervention.

- I see...
- Can you tell me more about that...
- It looks like this is hard to talk about...
- It sounds like you felt really angry, and also maybe a bit hurt, when he didn't come home that night?
- I know this may be painful, but can you tell me what happened next?
- And that made you feel better? Did that last?
- Let me see if I have this right; what you are saying is that it was the deception that most disturbed you?
- Hmm...
- What was going through your mind at that point?
- Imagine that things changed as you'd like... what would be different?
- That must have been pretty frightening...
- Wow...
- Sometimes when something like that happens people feel a certain satisfaction... was that true for you? Can you tell me a little about that...?
- And then you felt...?
- That's pretty normal...
- But...
- What about now? Do you still feel that way?

Figure 2-1. Worker statements that may prompt and reinforce client sharing, with particular emphasis on clarifying and communicating empathy with client emotions, clarifying the specifics of situations, or both.

Special Challenges

Why should the client trust you? Why should the client answer you honestly? Why tell you private information? Why follow through on collaboratively developed plans just because you indicate they may help? Unfortunately, many clients will appear resistant. It is crucial to recognize that clients have reasons not to engage, not to trust, and not to follow through that are rooted in their life experiences. Many clients have been severely disappointed by others all their lives; others have been disappointed by professionals many times. Many have never experienced an intimate relationship that was safe and predictable (see chapter 10 for further discussion of "personality disorders" and "disorders of the self"). In addition, the worker's behavior toward the client, particularly if it is experienced as punitive or coercive, is often a significant obstacle to developing an authentic collaboration.

Other difficulties arise when working with clients whose experiences differ significantly from those of the worker in terms of culture, ethnicity, social class, or any of the other dimensions that define our social world. Success in engaging under those circumstances depends on the worker's sensitivity, the worker's skills and knowledge of the cultures within which the client is embedded, the extent to which the worker has available a variety of repertoires that he or she can use differentially with different clients, and the client's readiness to accept services from someone who may be a member of a group with which the client has had negative experiences or who participates in negative equivalence relations.

Given such learning histories, it is often difficult to build a relationship with clients. It is the worker's responsibility to do so, not the client's. In this sense, "the client is always right"—if experience has taught the clients that others (or social workers specifically) cannot be trusted, the only way to change may be to have different experiences. Particularly with clients who are difficult to engage, the social worker will need to find ways to achieve the objectives discussed above (to communicate nonpunitive empathy, to find ways to reinforce, and to be seen as credible). Consistency despite challenges, creativity, nondefensiveness, and authenticity are helpful. The worker often must continue to act in these ways even as the client tests. Steps such as avoiding canceling or rescheduling appointments can be helpful to establish oneself as a predictable and reinforcing person.

Clinical Practice with Individuals

Supporting Health

In the context of the professional relationship, a subtle but crucial distinction exists between providing a nonpunitive audience and reinforcing pathology. Some professional helping may be damaging if it encourages clients to endlessly explore rather than act to change aversive situations, to dwell on unpleasant emotions rather than on taking the actions that will ultimately change them, or to produce increasingly bizarre verbalizations that the worker obviously finds fascinating. If the worker notices that the client continually and automatically repeats similar negative statements or seems to be searching for additional problems to discuss, this line may have been crossed. Once the client has told his or her story, much of the consultation time should be spent planning and acting to change the current situation, rather than dwelling on what is wrong. Feelings, of course, may not change quickly, and continued empathy for the client's feelings is always appropriate. Negative feelings, however, also should be seen as signals for the need to act differently (see chapter 4 regarding acceptance and commitment therapy).

The Clinical Session as a Sample of Behavior

The client's behavior during consultation with the social worker is probably best viewed as a genuine but limited sample of some forms of behavior that may occur elsewhere. Clients respond to social workers in ways that may be similar to how they respond to others (in the present or earlier in life). Sometimes a clinician has stimulus properties in common with others in the client's life history that may distort the client's reactions (the phenomenon called *transference*). Some related points should be kept in mind, however:

+ The ultimate purpose of consultation is to assist the client in constructing a fulfilling life, not to resolve the transference. If issues in the relationship are significant obstacles to achieving the client's goals, they are a legitimate focus of attention. However, the relationship is not an end in itself.

+ Human behavior is specific to the situation (Mischel, 1968), and it is often a mistake to assume that, for example, a man who seems thoughtful and perhaps a bit passive in the session could not possibly become enraged and beat his children. Some patterns of behavior generalize across multiple situations, but this is not always true. It is often necessary to collect data about what happens outside the session as well.

Given these caveats, the social worker's observations of how a client acts in the consultation session are useful data. For example, I recently saw a pregnant woman whose cohabiting boyfriend had left her after she became pregnant. She indicated that no family or friends seemed to be very supportive of her now and that they often seemed irritated with her. Achieving stronger social support was one of the areas she had established as a change goal. In her sessions, often when I would make an observation, she would find some part of what I said to qualify or disagree with (for example, "Well, not exactly . . ." or "No, not always"), even when the statement was clearly an accurate description or restatement of what she had just said. It seemed likely, and she later confirmed, that she often responded to people in that way, which of course punished others for speaking with her. In this case, learning to attend to points on which she could agree, in the session and outside, was an important repertoire to emphasize, a "clinically relevant behavior" (Kohlenberg & Tsai, 1991, p. 13).

In other cases, how the client describes himself or herself (for example, "I'm so stupid") may be characteristic of his or her self-talk at other times, and changing these verbal patterns may be an important treatment goal. In this case, the clinical emphasis should be not on punishing the client for making such statements (which would probably result in the client emitting them only covertly) but rather on collaboratively challenging the evidence for those statements as a way to modify the existing equivalence relation (me ≈ stupid) (Beck, Freeman, & Associates, 1990, called this process "collaborative empiricism"). Although the distinction may seem obvious, in practice it can be difficult to remember. The worker may find himself or herself merely challenging the client to stop speaking so negatively. This admonishment is probably not as effective as helping the client to identify situations that seem to support his or her "theory" and to examine whether what he or she does at those times proves he or she is "stupid"; it may also be helpful to identify situations in which the client clearly does not act "stupidly" and in the process perhaps construct more accurate equivalences.

Clinicians should maintain a dual focus, particularly during early exploration with clients, collecting the necessary information at the same time they are building relationships that encourage clients to provide that data (and later to experiment with sometimes uncomfortable change). The following material outlines core strategies for completing a broad but focused assessment from an ecobehavioral perspective; during this process, simultaneous attention to deepening the relationship is essential.

ECOBEHAVIORAL ASSESSMENT

Although some cases may be so straightforward that little assessment is required, most cases that occupy contemporary clinical social workers involve complex, transactional phenomena. Clinical work to address these cases requires collecting whatever data may be relevant and reaching an analytic understanding of what course would be required to attain the desired goal state. The following sections describe the five primary functions required in that process. Although the order in which they are described follows a certain logic (for example, looking in a comprehensive way at the case before deciding where to begin work), the assessment process in practice is seldom linear. The worker and client may circle back through these steps at several points in the case as circumstances change, as previously neglected pieces of information emerge, or in response to experiments undertaken by the client or the social worker. This nonlinear approach is to be expected, and a dynamic assessment of this sort provides far more guidance for intervention than would a static statement of what is wrong.

The five central functions required to complete an ecobehavioral assessment are (1) developing a vision of how the client's life could change, (2) conducting a broad, systemic ecobehavioral scan of the case in context, (3) extracting focal issues from that scan, (4) conducting behavioral analyses related to those issues, and (5) identifying interventive tasks that are responsive to that analysis (Mattaini, 1990). Notice that each step in this process is intimately and organically connected to those preceding and following it. For example, the behavioral analyses conducted in stage 4 should relate directly to the focal issues identified in the prior stage rather than to other areas identified in the broad scan. If the social worker loses sight of the connections, the work will become unfocused and ultimately ineffective.

Note that it is not only the behavior of the client that is being examined in this process, but also that of all of the actors (including, for example, family members and representatives of formal organizations) involved with the focal issues. Figure 2-2 is a sample interview guide tracing the identified stages. The reader may find it useful to refer to this guide while reading about each stage in the material that follows. This outline is meant only as a guide for conducting the assessment, not as a rigid questionnaire to be followed with every client in the same way. Different questions and emphases will be required in various practice settings and with each client. Questions such as these should be

I. Developing a preliminary vision.

- If we are successful, what is your vision of how your life will be different?
- Who will be doing what differently?
- Imagine that someone who doesn't know anything about you saw you when our work is complete; what would she actually see that is different from your life right now?
- When did this issue come up? How did it develop?

II. Ecobehavioral scan.

I'd like to ask you a few questions so I can understand your situation in the context of your everyday life. Let's try to develop a picture of what your life is like (you may wish to draw an ecomap during this stage or explore systemic transactions that may have relevance to the case, as suggested below).

- Let's start with what's right ... what areas of your life are currently going best for you?
- Who are the most important people in your life? (For first person identified:) How is that relationship? What's positive about it? How often do those positive things happen? On a scale of 0 (not at all) to 5 (a lot), how much satisfaction do you get from her? Are there also some struggles? How often do those come up? Same 0 to 5 scale, how much pain do those problems cause you?
- Who else (as above)?
- Does anyone else live in your home? How are your relationships with them? (For this and each of the following areas, inquire specifically about both positive and negative exchanges as necessary, and quantify.)
- What kind of contacts do you have with your extended family? Who else?
- Do you have many friends? How often do you see friends? How are those relationships? Anyone else?
- What about at work or school? What's going well there? So on our 0 to 5 scale ... Are there things that are not going too well? About a __ on our scale?
- Tell me a little about where you live. How satisfied are you with your home and your neighborhood?
- Do you have any religious or church affiliation? Are you active?
- Are you a member of any other groups or organizations?
- Any legal involvement?
- How is your physical health?
- How much do you drink? Do you take any medications or use any drugs?
- What would you like to do more of? What would you like to do less? (Suggest self-monitoring or observational measures to expand data.)
- What about emotions? Do you feel sad, tense, or angry very often? When does that happen? How long have you felt that way? (Pursue this further depending on responses; including use of self-anchored scales or rapid assessment instruments.)
- Are there any thoughts or images that disturb you? (Expand discussion as necessary.)

III. Extracting focal issues (contracting for change goals).

- So out of all of this, where do you think we should begin? What's most important to you?
- I notice that you seem to experience a fair amount of struggle with __. Is that something we should work on?
- What do you think would be a realistic goal here? Will that be satisfactory, or should we start somewhere else?
- Is there anything else we should work on at this point, do you think?
- So specifically, one of your goals is . . . (explicate in behavioral terms).

IV. Analysis of target behaviors.

Now, let's see if we can reach a clear understanding of your first goal or focal issue, which is . . . . (General flow is from current undesirable situation to goal state; this kind of analysis should occur for each identified target behavior, whether it is a behavior of the client, like angry outbursts, or of someone else, like a teenage child who is getting into trouble or a landlord who has not made repairs.)

- As near as you can tell, how did this problem start?
- When was that?
- Does this problem behavior ever pay off in any way for anyone—does it ever produce any advantages?
- Who or what supports the current behavior?
- What are the costs? What other problems does it cause?
- What seems to trigger the problem? Are there times when it doesn't happen? (Identify occasions.)
- Are there some times when this is not a problem? Tell me about those times . . . . When is the problem most likely to arise? (Search for motivating antecedents.)
- What do you think it would take to get from where you are to where you want to be? (Explore resources, including tangible, personal, and social)
- Who would be willing to help you achieve this goal or resolve this problem?
- Who or what might stand in the way?
- How important is this to you? Why? How will reaching this goal enrich your life? How quickly do you think that will happen? (Build motivation.)

V. Identification of interventive tasks.

(This part of the interview must be highly individualized. It should include exploration of possible interventive options for mobilizing the resources discussed in the previous section and for addressing obstacles identified, emphasizing approaches with the best empirical support within the realities of the case situation. Careful specification of the multiple steps required to work toward the goal is often required. Explore possible reinforcers to be used along the way as well.)

Figure 2-2. Sample interview guide. This is only a guide; not every question should be asked of every client. Areas that emerge as important to the case should be explored in-depth as needed, and the questions should be worked into the natural flow of the interview, during which the clinician is also working to authentically engage the client.

embedded in a natural clinical process that interweaves data collection and organization with furthering responses (for example, "Tell me more about . . .") and empathic responses (for example, "You sound very frustrated and maybe also pretty hurt about how your boyfriend has been spending his time.").

Developing a Preliminary Vision

The first question to be asked, although a complete answer often is not clarified until later in the process, is how the client would like to see his or her life change—a focus on the situation to be constructed, rather than on what is wrong. The advantages are twofold. First, constructing a vision of an improved life situation builds hope, whereas a primary focus on problems and pathology can be demoralizing. (The worker and the clinical situation also may come to participate in equivalence relations with "problems," making positive engagement more difficult.) The second advantage is strategic: Positive changes in the behavior of clients, collaterals, or others can be shaped and maintained through reinforcement, whereas a goal of eliminating behavior often requires relying on more punitive strategies.

Clients often think in terms of what is wrong, and the worker can start with that when it seems appropriate and then gradually shift the focus to how things might be different. In many cases, the client may be clear as to the general problem with which he or she is struggling; from this point, client and worker can move to envisioning positive alternatives. Even so, more data about the case situation are usually required to make a final collaborative determination of how to focus. For example, if a woman initially reports that she is depressed, but as she tells her story it becomes clear that she is being regularly and severely battered by a partner, the focus should shift to ways to ensure the safety of the client and to work to empower her (and perhaps to change the behavior of the batterer) rather than to general strategies for working with depression.

In other cases, clients may struggle to state even a first approximation of their hopes and concerns or may begin with something relatively unimportant and only later allow major issues to surface. I recently worked with a client who at intake asked for help because he felt anxious when reading and therefore was doing poorly in graduate courses. By the end of the interview, however, he had reported that he was involved in several sexual compulsions, including a variation of stalking; may have been sexually abused as a child; and was extremely isolated and lonely. As deeper and more central issues emerge, the focus of the interview should naturally shift to those.

Ecobehavioral Scan

Before deciding what to do, the worker should know what is happening in the client's world to understand the ecosystemic situation in which the client's life is embedded. I am using the term *ecobehavioral scan* here to emphasize that it is crucial to look at what actors are doing what (who is behaving in what ways) and at events and conditions that may prove to be involved in important contingencies. Many sources of data can be important in completing an adequate ecobehavioral scan. Clients themselves can accurately report the frequency with which problems occur and what the circumstances surrounding them may be. The clinical interview (structured as shown in Figure 2-2) is often the primary source of the data needed to complete the assessment, and the client clearly has access to information that no one else has. The interview can sometimes be wide-ranging, but it is important to focus limited available clinical time on areas that are central to addressing the principal issues in the case as they begin to emerge. It is not necessary or respectful to ask the client to share information not relevant to the purpose of the case (however interesting it may be). In many cases, and with the client's consent, data from collateral sources (for example, spouses, parents, employers, or agency representatives) can be collected through interviews. Not surprisingly, the more specific the data requested, the better information the social worker can get from such sources. Asking about specifics, in addition, may be helpful in prompting the collateral to notice both what the client does well and the problems.

During interviews the worker may determine that more detailed data will be valuable. Some behaviors can simply be counted, such as how many times a parent raises his voice to his child and how often his child did what she was told to do. Simple charts (often kept on the refrigerator or in a pocket) and counters (available in golf and sports stores) can add useful precision. Self-monitoring such as this sometimes has a beneficial effect by itself (for example, if you ask a person to count the number of positive statements he makes to his wife, the number may increase reactively in response to the client attending to this behavior). Clients report that self-monitoring can be empowering (Kopp, 1993), and it can also save limited clinical time. For example, one single mother reported that her four-year-old son was disobedient. When she kept track for a few days, however, she learned that her child did what he was told nearly all the time. Child compliance, therefore, despite the initial reports, did not become the focal issue in the case; rather decreasing mutual demands and increasing positive exchanges did.

The worker, or other staff or family members, also can directly observe and in some cases record client behavior. With a client who has severe mental illness, staff might count how many times the client makes delusional statements and graph this with data on visits from relatives. The data might show that the client does better during and after visits or might show the opposite; either would be important information for assessment. As another example, a client with a substance abuse problem may request or permit a spouse or significant other to provide data on substance use (which is sometimes more accurate than that provided by the client; see chapter 9).

Whole classes of behavior may be of interest. These classes of behavior can often be traced with behaviorally anchored rating scales (Daniels, 1994). For example, Figure 2-3 is such a scale designed by a social worker and her client to track his progress on making decisions—a relatively abstract behavior class (see Seidenfeld & Mattaini, in press, for a full report of the case).

A step less rigorous but still valuable is the use of simple self-anchored scales on which the client rates (for example, "on a scale of 1 to 10") how tense or sad or satisfied he or she feels. The mood thermometers (Tuckman, 1988), shown in Figure 2-4, include five such scales on a single instrument on which results can be graphed over time as has been done with data from a client of mine (Figure 2-5).

Another tool for combining multiple scales on a single image is the behavioral ecomap. One variety (shown in Figure 1-6 on p. 19) depicts the aggregate extent of reinforcers and aversives experienced by the client from other

Goal: To make timely and reasonable decisions based on analysis of probable consequences

Client fails to make or act on decisions—even when lack of action results in significant aversives	Client avoids acting on decisions until he experiences a high level of aversives for failing to act	Client is able to make and act on some decisions after someone else assists him to elaborate possible choices and clarify possible consequences for each; acts on choices only with substantial encouragement	Client independently identifies available choices and possible outcomes for each, and acts on this data under most circumstances with only limited additional support	Client regularly seeks opportunities to make choices, tracks consequences effectively, and readily takes reasonable risks to obtain valued reinforcement
-2	-1	0	1	2

Figure 2-3. A behaviorally anchored rating scale (BARS).

Clinical Practice with Individuals

How I Feel Right Now

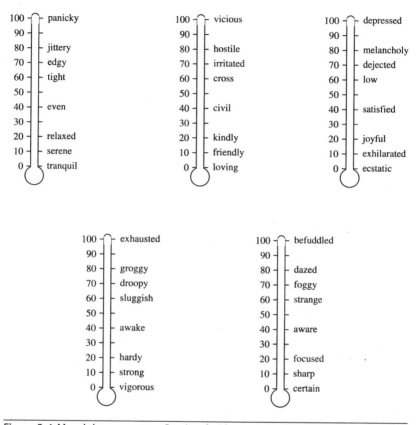

Figure 2-4. Mood thermometers. *Reprinted with permission from Ruckman, B.W.(1988). The scaling of mood.* Educational and Psychological Measurement, 48, p. 421. *Copyright 1988 by Sage Publications.*

people, entities, and the physical environment. Other varieties may be helpful in later stages of the assessment. One way to construct such an ecomap is to use client ratings on a self-anchored scale. The worker also can provide ratings, or the client and the worker can use the ecomap as an interviewing tool, discussing each area as exemplified in the interview guide (Figure 2-2) before filling in the diagram. For more precision, the data can come from an instrument such as the Community Interaction Checklist (Brown & Mattaini, 1996; Wahler, 1980; Panaccione & Wahler, 1986), which allows the client or worker to count the number or calculate the aggregate duration of various kinds of positive and negative exchanges experienced by the client.

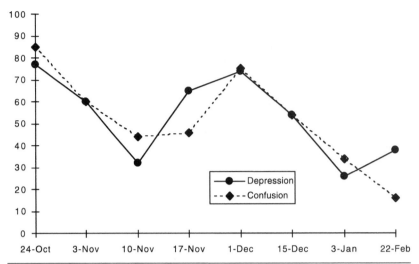

Figure 2-5. Scores on two of the mood thermometers (see Figure 2-4) for a 26-year-old client who presented initially with concerns about depression and confusion as well as dissatisfaction about the relationship with his girlfriend. Scores greater than 50 are in the undesirable range on each scale; those below 50 are in the desirable range. He ended that relationship in late November; note the spike in both depression and confusion around that time. The primary treatment approach was acceptance and commitment therapy (see chapter 4).

Sometimes it is valuable to capture data in detail over time. With some clients (those who are literate and have adequate record-keeping repertoires), the worker can ask the client to keep an hour-by-hour grid of his or her activities and level of satisfaction (or depression or tension or other emotion) while engaged in them. Actual client data for a depressed young woman are shown in Figure 2-6.

This tool allows the worker and client to trace the possible connections between environmental contingencies and emotional states. In the data shown, few periods occurred during which the client reported at least the subjective experience of much reinforcement from anywhere. Because depression was the focal issue, this deprivation clearly was important data. Experience suggests that most clients will keep this level of data reliably only for limited periods (one to two weeks at a time), although it can sometimes be repeated at intervals. If more data are needed, self-management strategies (see chapter 5) will usually be required.

As a part of the data collection process, social workers are increasingly turning to the use of standardized instruments, such as those included in the

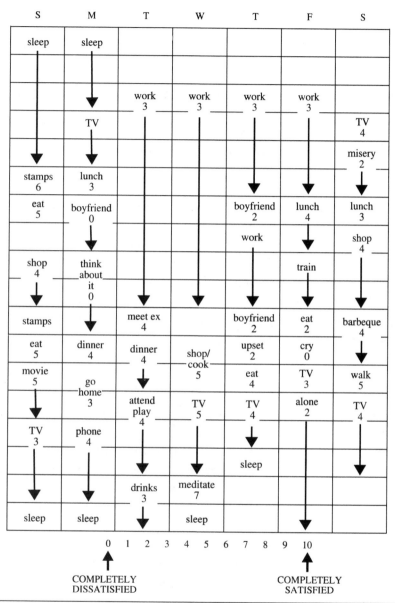

	S	M	T	W	T	F	S
	sleep	sleep					
		↓	work 3	work 3	work 3	work 3	
		TV					TV 4
	↓	↓					misery 2 ↓
	stamps 6	lunch 3			↓	↓	
	eat 5	boyfriend 0			boyfriend 2	lunch 4	lunch 3
		↓			work	↓	shop 4
	shop 4	think about it 0				train	
	↓	↓	↓	↓	↓	↓	↓
	stamps	↓	meet ex 4		boyfriend 2	eat 2	barbeque 4
	eat 5	dinner 4	dinner 4	shop/cook 5	upset 2	cry 0	↓
	movie 5	go home 3	↓	eat 4	TV 3	walk 5	
	↓	attend play 4	TV 5	TV 4	alone 2	TV 4	
	TV 3	phone 4	↓	↓	↓		
				sleep		↓	
	↓	↓	drinks 3	meditate 7			
	sleep	sleep	↓	sleep		↓	

0 1 2 3 4 5 6 7 8 9 10

↑ COMPLETELY DISSATISFIED ↑ COMPLETELY SATISFIED

Figure 2-6. A sample weekly activity grid showing varying levels of satisfaction over time.

Computer-Assisted Social Services package (Hudson, 1992). Hudson's system includes separate scales to measure the severity of problems such as depression, parent–child problems, and substance abuse (see Fischer and Corcoran, 1994, for a valuable collection of such instruments and an introduction to their use). When used by sophisticated practitioners who understand their limits with populations similar to those on which they have been normed, such instruments can be useful for gathering initial case data and for monitoring progress. At the same time, the limits of such instruments are significant, in part because they are usually only indirect measures of behavior. Although ecobehavioral social workers often use such instruments with clients, these practitioners nonetheless place more emphasis on behavior that can be directly observed or that the clients have monitored.

Extracting Focal Issues

By the time case data have been collected and conceptually organized, the core directions important to achieving the client's vision usually begin to emerge. These issues may involve repertoires to construct, increase, or decrease anywhere in the overall case configuration. There are several ways to determine where to start. Commonly, as the client tells his or her story and other data are collected as needed, certain crucial issues will become obvious. Often there will be a number of possible places to begin. When this occurs, there are several ways to decide on priorities. It may be necessary to address some problems quickly. Dealing with an eviction notice may be more emergent than deciding whether to go back to school. It may not be possible to resolve some issues until others are addressed; for example, clients often need to deal with active addictions before trying to reconnect with family estranged during years of substance abuse.

The clinical goals selected always involve behavior change of one kind or another. For example, the goal may be that parents and adolescent youths learn to communicate more effectively with each other. In other cases, the goal may involve the behavior of a system actor (for example, a landlord, an eligibility worker, or an absent father). In some cases, the core goal will relate to private events or conditions (such as depression). Even in these cases, change requires that one or more people act in a different way. For example, the social worker may provide new rules (an overt behavior) that the client then rehearses privately (covert behavior).

It is possible to focus on only a few change goals (probably no more than three in outpatient consultation) at once or the work is likely to become excessively diffuse. The worker and client can certainly decide to shift to new issues as the original foci are resolved or if conditions change, but this should be an explicit decision. Where possible, it may be best to begin with those

Clinical Practice with Individuals

issues on which some progress can be made quickly, turning to those that may be more difficult with some record of success.

Crucially, no matter what the worker may think should be addressed, unless he or she reaches an agreement with the client, substantive change is unlikely. This is as true for mandated clients as for those who are voluntary; some contract for what should be the focus of the work is universally required if clinical intervention is to result in lasting change. Clear agreement (even at an abstract level, such as "keeping you out of jail") may not be present in the beginning but should be a continuing focus of the work until the goal is achieved.

This stage of the assessment is also the moment to begin to determine how progress will be monitored. The basic question to be addressed is, "How will we know if things are getting better—whether the problems are being resolved or the goals reached?" Several of the approaches discussed above, such as counting and observing, self-monitoring, behaviorally anchored rating scales, or standardized instruments, are options here. Monitoring case progress is not some alien form of "research"; it is core to effective practice—how can we know progress is occurring if we do not know how to tell? It is critical to know whether progress is occurring, because lack of progress is a clear indication of the need to change the interventive plan, to re-examine the case to determine whether some important factor was missed during the assessment, or to examine whether a problem is occurring in the worker–client relationship that is blocking progress.

One approach to such monitoring that has particular usefulness in ecobehavioral practice is to combine the use of sequential behavioral ecomaps with a direct measure of the focal issue. For example, Figure 2-7 shows the quality and extent of social exchanges experienced by an initially insular single mother, along with measures of her use of positive reinforcement and punishment with her child. (The figure shows composite data, typical of one cluster of cases in a study with which I am involved. Available research suggests that insular parents who experience high levels of social coercion are less likely to have lasting positive outcomes from parent education as contrasted with those who experience substantial reinforcement from their social milieu [Panaccione & Wahler, 1986; Wahler, 1980]. The focal issue in this case is to increase the use of reinforcement and decrease the use of punishment, but the interventions may involve both teaching parenting skills as well as enriching the social network.)

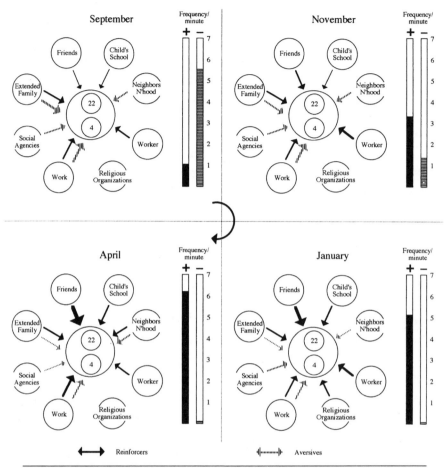

Figure 2-7. Sequential ecomaps portraying ecobehavioral transactions and frequency of positive reinforcement and punishment in parenting.

Once a small number of focal behavioral issues have been identified and restated if possible as behavioral goals, the next step is to complete an analysis of the contingencies within which the behaviors of interest are embedded. The more clearly the worker and client have clarified their goals, the easier it will be to move into the next stage. Ideally, at this point it is clear *who* the client wants to *do what* differently (self, family member, social contacts, agency staff, or others)—target behaviors have been specified.

Analysis of Target Behaviors

Many social work practice models emphasize the importance of completing an ecosystemic scan and identifying focal issues. Where the ecobehavioral model has the most distinct contribution to offer is in the fourth—analytic—stage of assessment. The central tasks at this stage are identifying contingency arrangements that may result in increases in identified goal behaviors or decreases in problem behaviors. In many cases it also may be valuable (or necessary) to understand contingencies active in maintaining the problem situation, although this is not true in all situations.

In one case the focal issue was increasing the rate of assertive behaviors by a 42-year-old client, Mitch, who tends to respond in many personal and professional situations in a relatively passive manner, until he becomes very frustrated. At that point, Mitch often becomes enraged and strikes out aggressively (except in situations—such as with his boss—when the risk of severe punishment is too high). As is always the case, we begin by looking at consequences. What consequences might help establish and maintain more assertive behavior on Mitch's part? A beginning analysis is shown in Figure 2-8.

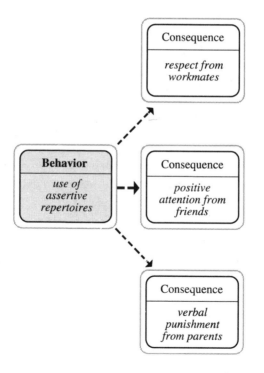

Figure 2-8. Consequences of use of newly acquired assertive repertoires.

Eventually, assertive behavior probably will produce better consequences from associates at work, from his girlfriend, and from his other friends. Discussion with Mitch suggested, however, that his parents were likely to punish assertive behavior toward them and even reports of assertion in other settings. The overall configuration suggests that Mitch's natural environment will ultimately provide enough reinforcement to maintain the new behavior. In the beginning, however, before he develops refined assertive skills and while others adjust to the change, he also may require extensive reinforcement from the social worker.

Antecedents are also relevant in this case. The social worker may provide rules for how to act more effectively and may offer models for Mitch to imitate in behavioral rehearsals. Appropriate occasions for using assertive skills will likely be provided by people at work, his girlfriend, and his friends. The presence of Mitch's parents, however, may become a signal that assertive behavior will not be reinforced, and he may rely on different repertoires with them than in other social situations.

Contingency diagrams can be used in similar ways, for example, to trace the contingencies associated with verbal aggression by an adolescent client at school. The upper panel in Figure 2-9 shows the contingencies associated with aggressive acts, whereas the lower panel shows those associated with complying with the demands of the school. Rather than simply labeling the client "aggressive," an image such as this enables the worker and client to understand the client's actions contextually. Clearly, multiple consequences are involved, as are powerful motivating antecedents and limited rule-governance repertoires. Contingency diagrams such as the one shown in Figure 2-9 enable the social worker to contrast the existing situation with the contingencies required to establish and support a new repertoire, as shown in Figure 2-10. Similar figures could be used to understand why a teacher acts punitively toward students rather than using positive reinforcers more extensively (see Mattaini, 1993, p. 245). The contingencies associated with the school administrator's acceptance of punitive discipline could also be explored in this way, as could those of members of the school board.

Two important concepts emerge from these last examples:
1. Clearly, the cultures within which the student in Figures 2-9 and 2-10 and the teacher described above are embedded are highly relevant to the issues and may need to be a focus of clinical attention if significant change is to be made.

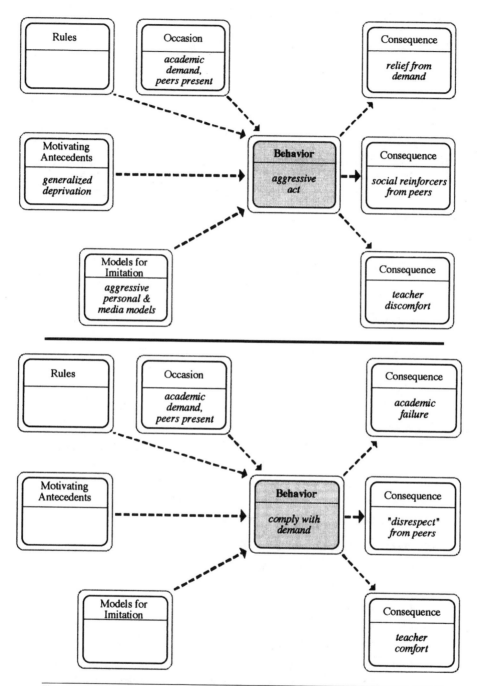

Figure 2-9. Contingencies associated with aggressive (upper panel) or compliant (lower panel) responses to academic demands, clarifying, for a particular adolescent, why the former is more likely than the latter. Blanks indicate areas of possible deficits.

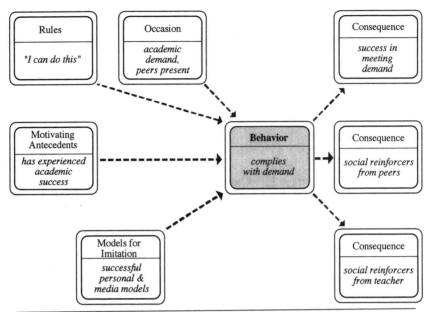

Figure 2-10. An alternative set of contingencies.

2. Examination of current contingencies is crucial. Personal history of consequences has shaped current problem behavior, but only different consequences from this point on (creating a new history) will ultimately change it. New antecedents of various kinds also may be required.

As the social worker begins physically or conceptually to sketch the clinical situation relevant to the focal issues in the case, he or she will often discover that there is missing information and that additional data are required to understand the problem. As before, such data can be gathered in multiple ways, including through interviews with client or collateral and by observation; such data collection may be required continuously or periodically throughout the consultation.

Identification of Specific Interventive Tasks

Multiple potential interventive options clearly emerge from the behavioral ecomaps or contingency diagrams shown in the figures. For example, if the client lacks the necessary repertoires or if no one provides much reinforcement for new efforts, meeting those needs become the tasks. If the problem behavior is maintained by attention, planned nonreinforcement may need to be arranged with the client's agreement. When the client does not have a clear view of the probable consequences, learning new rules may be useful. However, if the client clearly knows the rules but finds them hard to follow, self-management strategies may be required.

Many interventive task options are described in subsequent chapters; such tasks are selected precisely because they either involve direct changes in contingencies or may indirectly facilitate such changes. A social worker might help an isolated, depressed client to learn new self-talk and reinforce his or her increasingly assertive statements with the expectation that these skills will improve the client's social life. Alternatively, the worker and client might decide that he or she will experiment with joining several organizations, hoping that the social reinforcement available will provide some relief. Alternately, both approaches might be tried at once.

This approach is not mysterious. Once the contingencies have been identified (this is the professional challenge), the client can understand the situation as clearly as can the worker in most cases. This understanding can lead to a high level of client empowerment. To the extent possible, taking steps to change the active contingencies or to increase exposure to new ones should then be left to the client. In general, defining specific tasks to be achieved outside the session also advances the work, because it is usually contingencies outside the consulting situation that should be addressed.

Examination of a clinical situation will often show many possible points of intervention, and addressing all of them is not always realistic. The common environmental tenet "Think globally and act locally" has much to teach under those circumstances (Meyer, 1992). The challenge is to develop reasonable hypotheses about specific changes in consequences or antecedents that might substantially change the overall configuration. With some depressed clients, cognitive work might eventually lead to resolution of the problem, but a dramatic change in the client's social network may make changing his or her self-talk easier. In some cases, the resources required to make dramatic changes in contingencies may not be available, and the interventive task may be to increase the client's capacity for accepting a somewhat aversive situation. The clinical social worker should not move too quickly to this conclusion, however, because some change is nearly always possible.

DIAGNOSIS USING THE *DIAGNOSTIC AND STATISTICAL MANUAL OF MENTAL DISORDERS* AND THE PERSON-IN-ENVIRONMENT SYSTEM

Diagnosis, in the sense of mapping a client to one or more specific categories of disorder, is not a central feature of behavioral practice. Within this model, most problems are viewed as involving behaviors that are shaped and maintained by environmental contingencies, and most clinical issues are seen as transactional in nature, as the natural outcome of the client's experiences. Assigning a label to the client, rather than to the overall configuration over time, is inconsistent with this perspective. Many clinical issues are at least dimensional (from less to more) in nature, and most can be genuinely understood only when viewed in context. A diagnostic label often is not of substantial value for these purposes and can mislead the clinician into thinking he or she understands the problem, when in fact he or she would need to trace the relevant contingencies to do so (Mattaini & Kirk, 1991).

Familiarity with the American Psychiatric Association's (APA) *Diagnostic and Statistical Manual of Mental Disorders, Fourth Edition* (DSM-IV) (APA, 1994) is important, however, for several reasons. First, there are certain conditions—bipolar disorder, for example—that appear to be primarily rooted in biological malfunctions and for which medical interventions such as medication are required. (Even in such cases many other issues often are best viewed through an ecobehavioral lens. Refer to chapter 10 for more information.) Recognizing the possible presence of other diseases with organic roots is also important. Also, there are some learned patterns (such as panic disorder) for which specific interventive approaches have been empirically found to be particularly effective (see, for example, Barlow, 1993). In these cases, it is important to be able to determine whether the client's behavior generally fits the pattern of those for whom particular treatments have worked. So long as the clinical social worker also attends to the multiple ways that the environment has an impact on the client, familiarity with DSM diagnosis has its place.

The person-in-environment (PIE) social work system for diagnosing problems in role functioning and environmental problems is also available (Karls & Wandrei, 1994). In its current version, PIE does not capture connections among the behaviors of interest and the networks of interlocking contingencies in which they occur. Perhaps in a future version, this issue will be addressed. Given this limitation, PIE's primary usefulness now may be for statistical and reporting purposes, rather than for guiding interventive planning. It may prove valuable for program planning for an agency to know what proportion of its clients experiences problems with parenting or housing; the clinician, however, needs to assess the behavioral specifics unique to the case before guiding the client to a particular course of action.

CONCLUSION

This chapter has sketched the process of conducting a thorough ecobehavioral assessment that captures the transactional nature of case phenomena in an organic and holistic way. In fact, if an adequate assessment is made, the selection of interventions is often a relatively straightforward process. The following three chapters outline basic interventive strategies useful across a broad range of practice settings. Not every strategy is applicable to every case, but most clinical practitioners are likely to be able to use many of them at some point. I am using the term *strategy* here because interventions must be part of a coherent plan that emerges directly from the assessment and carefully tailored to the individual case. Ecobehavioral practice is not an unrelated bag of tricks but a coherent way of working with cases in context. It is particularly important that interventive techniques be organically embedded within the natural groups and networks to which the client belongs as determined by the assessment. This recognition is what makes ecobehavioral practice strategic in nature.

The material that follows is divided into three classes of interventive strategies. The first, covered in chapter 3 and the most powerful, is for the client and clinician to work directly with environmental contingencies. The second, discussed in chapter 4, deals with approaches for modifying private events, in particular emotional experiences (such as anxiety or depression), and self-talk (cognitive interventions). The third class of interventions (chapter 5) involves directly teaching the client new skills, such as assertive behaviors. The division is somewhat artificial because, for example, clients commonly need to change their self-talk before they are ready to take the risk of exposing themselves to new experiences. Many clients also may need to learn new skills before they can access new reinforcers. All of these connections should be clear if an adequate assessment has been completed.

REFERENCES

American Psychiatric Association. (1994). *Diagnostic and statistical manual of mental disorders* (4th ed.). Washington, DC: American Psychiatric Association.

Barlow, D. H. (Ed.). (1993). *Clinical handbook of psychological disorders* (2nd ed.). New York: Guilford Press.

Beck, A. T., Freeman, A., & Associates. (1990). *Cognitive therapy of personality disorders*. New York: Guilford Press.

Brown, E., & Mattaini, M. A. (1996, May 26). *Social coercion and parenting*. Paper presented at the meeting of the Association for Behavior Analysis: International, San Francisco.

Coady, N. F. (1993). The worker–client relationship revisited. *Families in Society, 74*, 291–298.

Daniels, A. C. (1994). *Bringing out the best in people*. New York: McGraw-Hill.

Fischer, J., & Corcoran, K. (1994). *Measures for clinical practice: A sourcebook* (2nd ed.). New York: Free Press.

Hudson, W. W. (1992). *WALMYR assessment scales scoring manual*. Tempe, AZ: WALMYR Publishing.

Karls, J. M., & Wandrei, K. E. (Eds.). (1994). *Person-in-environment system: The PIE classification system for social functioning problems*. Washington, DC: NASW Press.

Kohlenberg, R. J., & Tsai, M. (1991). *Functional analytic psychotherapy: Creating intense and curative therapeutic relationships*. New York: Plenum Press.

Kopp, J. (1993). Self-observation: An empowerment strategy in assessment. In J. B. Rauch (Ed.), *Assessment: A sourcebook for social work practice* (pp. 255–268). Milwaukee: Families International.

Lowery, C. T., & Mattaini, M. A. (1996). *The use of power in social work*. Unpublished manuscript.

Mattaini, M. A. (1990). Contextual behavior analysis in the assessment process. *Families in Society, 71*, 236–245.

Mattaini, M. A. (1993). *More than a thousand words: Graphics for clinical practice*. Washington, DC: NASW Press.

Mattaini, M. A., & Kirk, S. A. (1991). Assessing assessment in social work. *Social Work, 36*, 260–266.

Meyer, C. H. (1992). Social work assessment: Is there an empirical base? *Research on Social Work Practice, 2*, 297–305.

Mischel, W. (1968). *Personality and assessment*. New York: John Wiley & Sons.

Panaccione, V. F., & Wahler, R. G. (1986). Child behavior, maternal depression, and social coercion as factors in the quality of child care. *Journal of Abnormal Child Psychology, 14*, 263–278.

Seidenfeld, M., & Mattaini, M. A. (in press). Personal and family consultation services: An alternative to therapy. *Behavior and Social Issues*.

Skinner, B. F. (1989). The place of feeling in the analysis of behavior. In *Recent issues in the analysis of behavior* (pp. 3–11). Columbus, OH: Merrill.

Sue, S., & Zane, N. (1987). The role of culture and cultural techniques in psychotherapy. *American Psychologist, 42*, 37–45.

Tuckman, B. W. (1988). The scaling of mood. *Educational and Psychological Measurement, 48*, 419–427.

Wahler, R. G. (1980). The insular mother: Her problems in parent–child treatment. *Journal of Applied Behavior Analysis, 8*, 27–42.

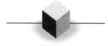

CHAPTER THREE

INTERVENTIVE STRATEGIES: EXPOSURE TO NEW EXPERIENCES

B ecause behavior is ultimately shaped and maintained by the contingencies within which it is embedded, the most powerful and direct route to
improving quality of life and changing behavior is exposure to different arrangements of environmental antecedents and consequences. Therefore, this
should be the primary social work interventive strategy—work with private
events and skills training as discussed in the next two chapters are adjunctive
procedures that can facilitate such exposure. Although many social work practitioners describe themselves as "ecologically oriented," this central core of
practice is often seriously underemphasized. Most adult clients can have a
major voice in deciding what new experiences to expose themselves to and
can take many of the steps required to do so. Action to change the contingencies that have substantial impact on oneself and recognition that one has the
capacity to do so are the defining features of personal empowerment.

There are two basic strategies for changing the individual's world in this
sense. First, it may be possible to embed new practices in cultures of which
the client is already a part. In work with a client whose spouse has a serious
problem with alcohol abuse, Thomas and his associates (Thomas, Santa,
Bronson, & Oyserman, 1987; Thomas & Yoshioka, 1989) have developed an
approach (see chapter 9) in which changes on the part of the client are likely
to induce changes in the spouse and ultimately reduce the level of mutual
coercion, struggle, and pain in the relationship as a whole. In this case, systemic changes are the result of new behavior by one member of the family.
Effective family work requires not only change in the behavior of one person
(although this may initiate a reciprocal process), but what Minuchin
(Minuchin, 1974; Minuchin & Nichols, 1993) calls "restructuring"—interlocking changes in family culture. In many social work cases, for reasons of

access, client readiness, or practicality, only one individual is seen. Even so, it is often possible to work toward embedding practices in the family (or other systems) that could help the client and family achieve their goals.

The second basic strategy is to expose the client to new webs of contingencies—new "cultures." For example, in contemporary life, many people drift into increasing isolation, resulting in significant loneliness and demoralization. Exposure to more opportunities to interact with people is important under such circumstances. Many supports may be required, including prompting and reinforcing from the clinician, teaching new skills, and changing client expectations (self-talk), but ultimately the goal is for the client to have new social experiences that work for him or her. If this happens, he or she is likely to continue to act in ways that result in more social contact. In one case, a male client in his early thirties worked with me for about one year to learn the skills needed to make and maintain a healthy primary relationship and manage an addictive behavior pattern. Finally, he was prepared to experiment with attending social functions and meeting women, at which point he made rapid progress because his new repertoires were richly reinforced.

Many other examples exist of how becoming a part of a new culture can be enormously helpful. For some clients, 12-step programs such as Alcoholics Anonymous are extremely valuable. An important active ingredient in such cases is probably the new networks of social reinforcement, including higher rates of reinforcement and reinforcement for behaviors consistent with maintaining sobriety. Another example is the Community Reinforcement Approach (see chapter 9) for work with substance abusers. This approach emphasizes changes in family culture and embedding the client in alternative vocational, recreational, and other networks, with the result that extensive reinforcement for remaining drug free is provided. Given what we know of the science of behavior, this is more likely to be effective than exhorting the client to "just say no."

In some cases, clients also may initiate or participate in the construction of new networks. A client who is a single mother with few social outlets may become involved with the worker in the development of a support group for women like herself or a play group for mothers and their children. Other clients may start their own businesses, leading to extensive changes in their social worlds.

Changing the networks of which the client is a part or connecting him or her with new ones is strongly emphasized in an ecobehavioral approach for two reasons. First, in significant numbers of cases, a major interventive goal is to help the client access higher levels of social reinforcement. The power of this strategy cannot be overemphasized. People are social entities, and a rich network of human connection can provide essential emotional and other supports, change one's definition of self, and reinforce healthy behavior. Second, behavior changes that the client undertakes often require substantial environmental support to be maintained. Although a good deal of consulting time is likely to be spent dealing with emotional experiences, changing self-talk, and building skills, most of this work is done to help the client achieve more effective connections with the social networks of which he or she is or wishes to be a part. Assisting the client to build positive connections and manage aversive ones is the core of clinical social work rather than an adjunct to treatment.

EXPERIMENTING WITH LIFE

Although the worker and client can often develop hypotheses about what a more fulfilling life may be like, the only way to be sure is to try it out, to "experiment with life." What kind of experiment to try is often suggested by the assessment. For example, a socially anxious and isolated client in his late twenties wished to build relationships with women, an area in which he had only limited experience. Although he could identify several available women he might be interested in dating, actually dating them felt like too large a step for him in the beginning. So he and the social worker made a list of things he might try as first steps. He decided that he could begin by having an informal conversation at least once a week with any of several women at work and that (somewhat surprisingly) he wanted to take dancing lessons. He was able to do the first after rehearsing conversational openings and what he might talk about with each. He was able to do the latter after planning ways to deal with probable obstacles that could arise; this is a good example of trusting the clients' judgments of their readiness to take action. Given these early successes, the client then began making plans to return to school for further education (a setting in which he would also have more social contact) and to explore becoming more involved in church organizations.

Clients also can experiment with introducing new variations into the existing cultures of which they are members. This is a common approach for improving transactions in families, but similar strategies can be used in other settings. A client reported that she hated her job because staff morale in the human services agency where she worked was poor, and people often were aversive to each other as well as to clients. In the course of consultation, she decided there were two approaches she might try: organizing a "morale committee" to plan special staff events and making a specific effort to increase the level of positive reinforcement exchanged in the agency. To do the latter, she developed a self-monitoring plan in which she kept track of the number of times she gave sincere recognition for a good idea or a job well done to other members of the staff, graphed those events, and then gradually set higher criterion levels for herself. There were two positive outcomes: the client certainly felt more empowered to act to change her world by taking these steps and she believed (although she did not specifically measure this) that her efforts had made a noticeable change in the organizational culture.

Experiments may involve introducing changes into the client's microculture. In work with a member of a couple one way to improve the quality of the relationship may be for the client to hypothesize actions or events the other partner might appreciate and try implementing some of those, at first unilaterally. The other partner may then be more responsive in turn (case data collected by my colleagues and me as well as some harder research [Bornstein, Anton, Harowski, Weltzien, McIntyre, & Hocker, 1981; Bornstein, Hickey, Schulein, Fox, & Scollati, 1983] suggest that positive reinforcement tends to be reciprocated, as are aversives, in intimate relationships). This strategy may not be effective in every case, given differences in individual learning histories, so this kind of intervention should be treated as an experiment. In some families, it may be important to offer reinforcers contingent on desired behavior; in others, to simply provide a higher overall rate (see chapter 8 for further detail).

Not every effort clients attempt will succeed, of course. By framing these tasks as experiments, the client can return to the social worker, problem solve about what went wrong, and then design new experiments to test, without describing their efforts or themselves as failures. Although not every scientific experiment works, something can be learned from each; the same is true of life experiments.

FIXED-ROLE THERAPY

Another form of experiment that can be useful is an updated version of fixed-role therapy, which Kelly presented more than 40 years ago (1955/1991). In

Clinical Practice with Individuals

this approach, the client and clinician imagine the client acting in a very different way than he or she usually does, as if playing a part in a play or taking on a new "role." The new role may be modeled after an admired person or may be an aggregate of traits of several people. The use of models is not essential but may be helpful in fleshing out the new repertoires that the client wishes to test. Kelly and his colleagues found that a major change was easier for people to maintain than small adjustments, which makes theoretical sense from an ecobehavioral perspective because the consequences of a major change are likely to be substantially different.

The client and worker, after developing the new role and perhaps role playing it in session, determine when and for how long the client will try living the new role in his or her life. Role playing may be applicable in only one of the cultural networks within which the client acts, such as at work, or it may be more generalized. For example, a passive client may decide to go into several stores and play the part of an assertive person, modeling his behavior after that of a friend, or a man who tends to be undemonstrative in relationships may decide to spend one day acting like a character in a movie who is emotive and overtly sensitive. Before taking on these tasks, it is important that the client be aware of the relevant actions and have them in his or her repertoire. One approach is to have the client list the specific behaviors that the new role involves and to flesh these out through discussion and rehearsal; another is to try to act exactly as the identified model would in various circumstances.

The intent of this approach is not necessarily for the client to take on the new persona permanently, although some clients may choose to do so. Rather, it is to experience that acting differently produces different social consequences and that one has options in terms of how one acts and therefore what kind of reactions one receives. These can be empowering experiments, because they may give the client an enhanced recognition of the extent to which he or she can act to change his or her social world. Whether or not the outcome is satisfying, the effort will produce useful data for planning how to proceed. The use of fixed-role therapy is probably indicated when clients seem clear about how they would like to be able to act but have not yet been able to do so. If anxiety is one dimension of the case, which it often is, it may make sense to begin by experimenting in less-threatening settings and then to move gradually to progressively more challenging ones.

DESIGNING EXPERIMENTS

The client and worker have several approaches to decide what experiments to try. In the assessment interview, as discussed in the previous chapter, one of the most critical areas is envisioning the goal, specifically how the client's life would be different if intervention is successful. Once this is established, setting subgoals is useful, and client tasks often will involve taking first steps toward those goals or taking actions that are similar to those they ultimately hope to take but are perhaps less anxiety producing. For example, a socially anxious client may commit at first to attending structured social events where he or she may not be required to be very active.

The process of designing experiments should begin early in the clinical consultation, preferably in the first session. Deciding on specific experiments to attempt and designing them in collaboration with the client may require the social worker's best analytic and relationship skills. It is best to begin with the client's vision of an enhanced future and determine what could be done immediately that could be a small step toward that. If the client wants ultimately to have a richer social life but is currently nearly immobilized by anxiety, deciding to spend a few minutes several times in the next few days in a public setting where many people congregate may be a first step (exposure is the most effective intervention for many anxiety problems); perhaps this step could then be followed by involvement in a structured social situation such as a church meeting. A first step for a person who experiences few positives in life may be to work on a list of possibly positive experiences and then try the easiest experience (see chapter 7 for details). If the issue relates to an unsatisfying relationship, the client may try acting differently in the relationship (chapter 8) or spend more (or less) time with the person involved.

The first experiments should be easy to complete; early success can build commitment for more difficult later steps. Once the basic plan is determined, Reid's task planning and implementation sequence (Reid, 1992) can be useful for ensuring a positive experience. The following are the steps involved in this sequence:

+ generating alternatives
+ establishing motivation
+ planning details of implementation
+ anticipating obstacles
+ doing guided practice, rehearsal

- agreeing on tasks
- summarizing.

The worker must, if an experiment has been developed in one session, discuss the outcome of the experiment in the following session (or between sessions by phone if necessary) to emphasize how essential such experiments are for achieving a successful clinical outcome. It is often useful to write down the tasks planned and to keep one copy for review in the next session.

REFERENCES

Bornstein, P. H., Anton, B., Harowski, K. J., Weltzien, R. T., McIntyre, T. J., & Hocker, J. (1981). Behavioral-communications treatment of marital discord: Positive behaviors. *Behavioral Counseling Quarterly, 1,* 189–201.

Bornstein, P. H., Hickey, J. S., Schulein, M. J., Fox, S. G., & Scolatti, M. J. (1983). Behavioral communications treatment of marital interaction: Negative behaviors. *British Journal of Clinical Psychology, 22,* 41–48.

Kelly, G. A. (1991). *The psychology of personal constructs: Vol. 1—A theory of personality.* London: Routledge & Kegan Paul. (Original work published 1955)

Minuchin, S. (1974). *Families and family therapy.* Cambridge, MA: Harvard University Press.

Minuchin, S., & Nichols, M. P. (1993). *Family healing.* New York: Free Press.

Reid, W. J. (1992). *Task strategies.* New York: Columbia University Press.

Thomas, E. J., Santa, C., Bronson, D., & Oyserman, D. (1987). Unilateral family therapy with the spouses of alcoholics. *Journal of Social Service Research, 10*(2–4), 145–162.

Thomas, E. J., & Yoshioka, M. R. (1989). Spouse interventive confrontations in unilateral family therapy for alcohol abuse. *Social Casework, 70,* 340–347.

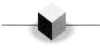

CHAPTER FOUR

INTERVENTIVE STRATEGIES: WORK WITH COGNITIVE AND OTHER PRIVATE EVENTS

F eelings and thoughts, although not directly observable to others, are behavior and are often central foci in clinical practice. Clients are unlikely
to take the risks to expose themselves to new situations if they say to themselves, "This will never work," or if visualizing a change leads to severe anxiety
and panic. Not only are thoughts and feelings significant in direct work with
clients, they also are relevant to work with significant others or collaterals. If
a teacher believes that all single mothers on welfare are lazy and do not care
about their children, he or she is less likely to be responsive if a single mother
receiving welfare visits the school to discuss the child's progress. Clinical work
often involves intervening in the cognitive or emotive modalities with the
client directly or with others within the boundaries of the case.

A number of different treatment approaches for work with thoughts and
feelings are available. For example, rational-emotive behavior therapy, as developed by Albert Ellis (Ellis & Whitely, 1979; Yankura & Dryden, 1990),
and cognitive therapy, as exemplified by the work of Aaron Beck (Beck, Rush,
Shaw, & Emery, 1978; Beck, Freeman, & Associates, 1990), are effective approaches for changing problematic self-talk. Many approaches, from Gestalt
therapy to acceptance and commitment therapy (ACT), have been developed for work with private events. It is critical, however, that the clinical social worker not just draw randomly from these approaches but rather view
cases as coherent, integrated wholes. If ecobehavioral assessment indicates
that thoughts or emotions are significant obstacles to an enriched and more
fulfilling life for the client, these may become focal issues for work. Changing
these thoughts depends on identifying the events and conditions that have
shaped and maintained them and on arranging new contingencies that will
support alternatives.

This chapter discusses several interventive strategies for work with private events. The four basic strategies presented are choices and consequences, changing self-talk, ACT, and exposure. The first two strategies draw extensively from the work of cognitive–behavioral therapists, whereas ACT and exposure are primarily behavioral in nature. These techniques are presented not as a random "bag of tricks" but rather as strategies that fit organically within an ecobehavioral practice approach to be used when they are consistent with an overall analytic understanding of the case. Although they are presented separately and sequentially here for clarity, it is common to integrate elements from several of these strategies in work with a case. For example, in cases of debilitating anxiety, it is common to combine exposure with changing self-talk; in problem solving using choices and consequences, acceptance also is often important.

CHOICES AND CONSEQUENCES

The phrase *choices and consequences* is a simple one suggested by a number of theorists of different orientations, but it is used in a specific manner here. The basic concept is easily accessible to clients. As many clients describe their difficulties, the clinician will be aware that the repertoires of clients are weak with regard to being aware of multiple options in problem situations, being able to project probable short- and long-term consequences of each, and acting based on these observations. These observational, verbal, and overt behavioral skills are those that are often presented as problem solving (Goldfried & Davison, 1976; Reid, 1985). Common models for problem solving include a variable number of steps but usually include specifying the problem, identifying and evaluating alternative responses, acting on the best available response, and evaluating the outcome.

In ecobehavioral practice, the skills required can be clearly specified. First, in a challenging situation (one in which there is high level of aversives or an inadequate level of reinforcers), clients need to learn that there are usually multiple options (a rule). Second, they then need to learn to describe the possible options and probable consequences of each. This ability to accurately describe aspects of reality is a critical skill—although the worker can initially model it for clients, learning to do so independently is important for long-term client satisfaction. Third, clients need to learn to act based on the consequences they have identified. Although it may seem that this would happen automatically, being aware of and able to describe contingencies is different from following the resulting rules. For example, one social worker of whom I am aware conducted HIV prevention groups for adolescents in which she emphasized the importance of using condoms if one chooses to have sexual intercourse and taught the necessary practical and interpersonal skills to do so. However, the social worker often had unprotected sex with multiple partners. Theoretically, this is understandable, because describing (*tacting*) contingencies and modifying one's behavior based on the rules so extracted (*tracking*) are different repertoires (Hayes, Zettle, & Rosenfarb, 1989). Developing such skills requires learning to describe choices and consequences and committing to taking the actions suggested, at first perhaps only with substantial encouragement and reinforcement from the social worker. Gradually, the worker can then decrease his or her involvement as the client comes increasingly under the control of natural contingencies. This represents movement from pliance to tracking (Hayes, Zettle, & Rosenfarb, 1989).

The analysis above is more technical than what most clients need. Learning to identify choices and to project, plan, and act based on likely consequences is usually adequate. For example, a client who is trying to decide the next step to take in a romantic relationship—whether to marry, to end the relationship, to spend some time apart, or to continue the present arrangement for a while before making any decision—should learn first that these (and perhaps variations of each) are his or her choices. The worker may need to assist the client in identifying these choices, often by using a Socratic questioning approach (for example, "Are those the only choices you see? Perhaps there are others that are less final?"). It is valuable, however, not only to assist the client to identify options and alternatives but also to help him or her to be aware that is what he or she is doing. In this way, it is more likely that a generalized repertoire of identifying multiple available choices in a variety of challenging situations will develop. The best available choice, of course, is not always ideal. A homeless client may need to decide on a bitterly cold night whether to try to survive outdoors or go to a shelter where he or she does not feel safe. The choices and consequences strategy, however, is still useful in such situations.

One important component of the choices and consequences strategy is learning to describe the multiple positive and negative short- and long-term consequences for each alternative. The clinician can ask questions and make

Clinical Practice with Individuals

comments such as the following to begin to shape this repertoire: "What are your choices?" "Are there others?" "Let's think wildly for a minute; I suppose you could . . ." "What would be the immediate payoffs if you did that?" and "If you did that, what would happen in the long run?" Although asking questions such as these in a free-form way may be adequate, it is important to label the process (for example, as choices and consequences) to help the client see the equivalences among multiple situations in which the strategy is relevant. It also may help to complete a matrix such as the one shown in Figure 4-1 to ensure that the client–worker team considers all likely consequences of each realistic option.

Identifying the consequences of multiple options is one component of acting to obtain the best possible set of consequences, but it does not ensure that clients will do so, for several reasons. First, learning to act based on probable real-world contingencies (tracking) is a skill that requires practice. Second, learning to work for a better-quality or larger reinforcer that is delayed, as opposed to a poorer-quality immediate payoff, is a challenging rule-governed repertoire, particularly if the immediate contingencies are strong. For example, a gay man who believes he will be better off in the long run if he leaves an emotionally abusive relationship may find the immediate guilt produced by taking steps out of the relationship a powerful aversive. Another client may believe that completing high school would be valuable, but the immediate distracting contingencies provided by nonattending friends and aversives imposed by a difficult teacher may make regular attendance difficult.

Choice	Positive Short-term Consequences	Negative Short-term Consequences	Positive Long-term Consequences	Negative Long-term Consequences
1.				
2.				
3.				
4.				
5.				
6.				

Figure 4-1. A choices and consequences matrix.

Interventive Strategies: Work with Cognitive and Other Private Events

Several strategies may be useful under such circumstances. A particularly valuable one is the use of self-monitoring and self-management strategies, discussed in chapter 5. Another approach (appropriate in only some circumstances) is for the worker to assist the client to develop rules and then provide social reinforcement for the desired behavior in the beginning, gradually fading these artificial contingencies as natural ones take over. An inspirational and deeply caring social worker can often provide the encouragement needed for the client to take difficult steps. Ultimately the goal is to reach the point at which the natural contingencies can support the new repertoire. If this expectation cannot be arranged, the established goal may be unrealistic.

Many clients are ambivalent when faced with difficult choices (particularly when each is to some extent aversive). Several approaches are useful for working with ambivalence. First, completing a choices and consequences matrix such as the one shown in Figure 4-1 may help to clarify the competing contingencies. Second, with issues that are not extremely important, it may be useful to point out to the client that making any of several reasonable choices may be better than staying stuck, particularly when this can be done experimentally. It may matter less which high school program a client decides to attend than that he or she attends one of them. Finally, when ambivalence is high, it is often best to try the least final alternative first. A client in an unhappy primary relationship may identify her choices as trying to induce her partner to enter couples counseling or leaving. If she is very uncertain, the first may be the best place to start.

CHANGING SELF-TALK

Cognitive therapy emphasizes changing self-talk—what clients say to themselves (often covertly). Several kinds of self-talk can cause difficulties. One class consists of inaccurate rules. For example, a client may, based on one or a few experiences, overgeneralize that, "No matter what I do, no one likes me." If the client also has learned a rule saying, roughly, "It is critical that everyone like me," the stage is set for emotional upset. Some cognitive theorists suggest that such evaluations are always mediating factors between external events and emotional responses. This understanding is probably oversimplified. Current evidence suggests that in some cases self-talk occurs before the emotion is experienced; in other cases the emotion occurs first followed by self-talk. In some cases of emotional upset, there may be little cognitive involvement at all (Kohlenberg & Tsai, 1991). Still, it appears clear that in many cases changing self-talk can change emotional reactions as well as facilitate more overt action. Another variety of problems related to inappropriate rule governance is, in a sense, the opposite of the sort of problem addressed by choices and consequences (in which rule-governed repertoires are too weak). Some clients are excessively rule bound and therefore are not adequately sensitive to contingencies. For example, some clients may observe themselves critically in social situations, watching for moments when they do something "awkward" and then punishing themselves when that occurs.

A second major type of problematic self-talk relates to problematic equivalence relations. A client who has learned the equivalence

$$me \approx foolish \approx stupid \approx unpopular$$

is likely to suffer from what has popularly (and too loosely) been labeled "low self-esteem." Different interventive strategies are needed for each of these types of issues.

Changing Inaccurate Rules

Cognitive therapists have identified many inaccurate rules, and particular clients often have learned idiosyncratic ones. Some types of self-talk are common, however; Figure 4-2 lists some of these with examples. In some cases, the origin of these kinds of self-talk may be clear. Some clients, for example, report that they can still hear their parents warning them that, "You can't trust anyone" (overgeneralization), or saying, "This is a disaster" when something goes wrong ("awfulizing" in Albert Ellis's colorful language). Others no doubt have learned such inaccurate rules through other life experiences. It is seldom important and often impossible to identify the source of such rules; what is important is to change them. Much problematic self-talk consists of fragmentary rules. Although the complete rule may be something such as, "No matter what I do, terrible things will happen to me," the actual words the person says to himself or herself may be something like, "Why bother?" Clinically, it is often useful to help the client spell out the complete rule, which can then be tested.

Some cognitive therapists believe that there are two levels of cognitive events: automatic thoughts (roughly what I am calling self-talk) and underlying schemas (more general patterns). It may be clinically useful to think about the second as either functionally equivalent classes of self-talk, any of which may appear under similar conditions, or classes of self-talk that have generalized to a range of

Overgeneralizing
- Nothing I do ever comes out right.
- You can never trust anyone.
- Everyone else is always happy, but I never am.
- Everything always goes wrong for me.
- No one does, or ever will, care about me.
- I am weak; I cannot deal with problems on my own.

Selective Attention, Exaggeration (Idealizing, "Awfulizing"*)
- You are perfect in every way.
- This is a disaster, it's just awful.
- If someone is upset with me, it's terrible.
- I am the smartest, best-looking, most thoughtful person around.
- I made a mistake, so I'm obviously a complete failure.
- If I don't find a spouse, my life will be a total waste.
- I can't stand this.

Placing Excessively Rigid Demands on Self or Others
- I must do everything perfectly.
- You must do what I want you to, or you don't care about me.
- I should be able to keep everyone happy all the time.
- No one has a right to do things that I don't like.

* The term "awfulizing" was introduced by Albert Ellis.

Figure 4-2. A sampling of inaccurate self-talk.

different conditions, rather than as some sort of hypothesized mental structures. In other words, the focus is on cognitive events, viewed as processes, instead of on structures. (From either perspective, the way self-talk or hypothetical schemas are changed involves work directly with self-talk.)

Two distinct approaches exist for changing self-statements, although the two blend into each other in practice. The first is a process called *rational disputation*, gently confronting clients with evidence that their current self-talk is not consistent with reality and helping them to practice alternative self-statements. If a client indicates that "It would be awful if I got turned down by Harvard!" the worker might say, "Imagine for a minute that you don't get accepted. Would that really be *awful*? Would it mean you are a worthless person? That your life is over?" with the intention that the client will see the irrationality and exaggeration in his or her thinking. This sort of confrontation can often be done with considerable humor; the more engaged clients are and the more they see the social worker as knowledgeable, the more confrontation of this sort they are likely to be able to tolerate. Once the current thinking is seen as clearly irrational, the worker can help the client formulate more realistic self-statements. For example, a client who tends to tell himself or herself that it is important that everyone approve of everything he or she does might practice alternatives such as, "I would prefer it if everyone always liked what I do, but of course they won't. And I can live with that."

Rational disputation is often associated with Albert Ellis (Ellis & Whitely, 1979; Yankura & Dryden, 1990), whereas the second basic strategy for changing self-talk, collaborative empiricism, was described originally by Aaron Beck (Beck, Rush, Shaw, & Emery, 1978; Beck, Freeman, & Associates, 1990). Rather than confronting the client with evidence of inaccurate self-talk, in collaborative empiricism the worker and client develop experiments to test whether self-statements are accurate. For example, a dialogue between a social worker and a depressed teenager might go as follows:

Client: My mother is completely disgusted with me since I got Bs and Cs on my last report card. She had her heart set on my getting a full-tuition scholarship to college since she can't afford to send me, and now I'll never even get in.

Worker: What makes you think she is completely disgusted with you? How sure are you about that?

Client: I'm pretty sure.

Worker: José, would you be willing to try an experiment? Could you ask your mother?

Client: Maybe . . . I don't know how to bring it up, though.

Worker: OK! Let's practice how you might ask; then you can decide.

In this exchange, the worker might begin with a focus on the client's interpretation of what his mother was thinking, or perhaps on the probably exaggerated importance being placed on a single report card, or on each in turn. In the dialogue, the worker did not challenge the client, but rather simply asked for data. He or she also gave a clear message in the final line that, ultimately, the decision about whether to go ahead with the experiment was the client's, a respectful and empowering stance.

In the beginning, clients will often agree that alternative ways of thinking are more sensible but will say they do not feel it yet emotionally. What this really means is that they need to act in terms of the new rules, and experience the actual consequences, before emotional (visceral) reactions will change.

Self-talk is like any other behavior—it must be practiced, often under a variety of circumstances, before it becomes automatic. In the meantime, it may feel alien, particularly because many situations have become associated with the old way of thinking. The solution is to practice, preferably often. One valuable approach is to have the client keep a self-talk log (Figure 4-3) between sessions. The log provides practice as well as considerable valuable data about the circumstances when problematic self-talk occurs. It can also be useful to arrange small reminders (for example, a small piece of colored tape on the face of one's watch or a sticker on the bathroom mirror) to remind oneself to practice new self-talk. These reminders may need to be moved or changed regularly so the client does not get so used to seeing the prompt that he or she no longer pays attention.

Decreasing Excessive Rule Governance

Many clients are seen in part because they constantly scan to make sure they do not make any mistakes ("I must please everyone," "I shouldn't waste time") and as a result make themselves miserable. They are rule bound and as a result miss many of the direct-acting reinforcers that they either are or might be exposed

Describe the Situation	Inaccurate Self-Talk	Accurate Self-Talk
Saturday night, 9 p.m., I am at home alone.	I will never be able to find a romantic partner, and if I don't, I will be miserable forever. (overgeneralizing, awfulizing)	I really would like to find a romantic partner, and there may be things I can do to make it more likely. But if I don't, I can find other pleasures in life.
Monday, 11 a.m., my boss calls me into the office and angrily points out a mistake I made on a report.	I am a complete screw-up; I can never do anything right, and I'm sure I'll be fired any time now. (excessive demandingness, awfulizing)	I wish I hadn't made that mistake; I should think of a plan to prevent this in the future. I usually do good work, though, so my boss will probably get over this.
Tuesday evening, my sister calls and says she can't make it to my party on Saturday night. I have been planning this party for months and was really counting on her help.	She is such an uncaring, ungrateful person, I will never speak to her again. She doesn't give a damn about me. (overgeneralizing, excessive demandingness)	I was really hoping she would help me with this, and I'm really disappointed. I may not always be able to count on her, but she has often done things for me in the past.

Figure 4-3. A sample self-talk log.

to. In contrast to the client whose behavior is inadequately governed by rules and who may appear impulsive (for whom choices and consequences may be valuable), the behavior of these clients may largely occur to avoid guilt and embarrassment. As a result, they may avoid taking even minimal risks that may be required to enrich their lives. To resolve this issue, clients must take risks often enough to experience the advantages. Clinicians can assist such clients by prompting them to take small risks at first and by reinforcing any effort at spontaneity in the beginning (even if the results are mixed because of lack of skill); these steps are a special case of exposure, which is discussed later in this chapter. However, attention to clients' self-talk during such exercises also may be useful, teaching them to listen to what they are telling themselves ("she might say 'no'; that would be so embarrassing") and practicing alternatives ("She might say 'yes'; that would be great. She might say 'no,' and I might feel embarrassed, but I can live with that, and it's worth the risk"). Note that in the second example, the client does not try to deny or fight the *feeling*—that is accepted, but experiencing the feeling is normalized, not awfulized. The value of this (and other) forms of acceptance is a core principle of acceptance and commitment therapy, which is discussed in a later section.

Changing Equivalence Relations

One of the areas examined in conducting an initial and ongoing case assessment relates to identifying problems with equivalence relations. This identification may include those relations in which the person associates himself or herself with negative events, attributes, or conditions (for example, [myself ≈ fat ≈ ugly]) or other overgeneralized and inaccurate classes, such as [people ≈ selfish ≈ cold]. This is another form of problematic self-talk: problem associations among antecedents, behaviors, and consequences that have been established by unfortunate experiences. An emotionally abusive parent might respond to a child's report that she won a contest in school by saying, "Jane! You? Your teacher must have been drinking; you couldn't have won!" At a time when she is angry, the parent may call Jane "stupid." As a result of many such experiences, the child is likely to develop equivalence relations such as me ≈ stupid ≈ incompetent, and as a result, when she thinks of herself or sees herself in the mirror, other elements of the relation are likely to emerge. Ultimately, an equivalence relation is not a thing or a structure; rather, in the presence of one image or word, another is likely to be produced. For example, the word "fool" evokes the word "me"; the word "death" evokes the word "release"; or the presence of a person of color evokes the word "dangerous." Inaccurate equivalences can result in overgeneralization or in completely erroneous associations.

This is a technical discussion, but it is important to understand the underlying process to intervene effectively. Changing rules and equivalence relations can be difficult because both can be insensitive to immediate contingencies. Some clinicians have suggested that one way to change problematic equivalence relations may be the use of paradoxical interventions (Dougher & Hackbert, 1994) (for example, "It's good you are confused"), but paradox can seem noncollaborative unless the reason for taking that direction is explained.

Although research in this area is in its infancy, it appears to be possible to teach new relations, and the goal of the clinician–client team may be to do so explicitly through practice and reinforcement. The worker may say, for example, "Do you notice how often you say 'I'm such a screw-up' and 'There I go again' and 'I always end up embarrassing myself'? You seem to say those things so automatically! I wonder how true they are [notice that here the clinician is using a bit of collaborative empiricism]. Do you really screw *everything* up? . . . [discussion] . . . Could it be that you are just a more spontaneous person, who doesn't worry so much about image all the time?" The goal in such discussions is to form new relations, for example, [me ≈ spontaneous ≈ honest], and to some extent to reverse the existing classes, changing [me ≈ dumb] to [me ≈ smart] in many ways.

Logs and written assignments may be helpful here (logs and assignments similar to those used when changing inaccurate rules). Clients are asked to note the evidence when they make negative self-appraisals and to practice more accurate statements. As in parenting, in which it works better to pay attention to specific successes and positive behaviors on the part of the child than to vaguely say, "You are a good boy," it is also usually best for clients to try to avoid global judgments of themselves (good person/bad person) and attend to specific effective or ineffective behaviors. Still, if a person is told often enough, "That was a mean thing to do" or "You were really cruel to her," a relation such as [me ≈ mean ≈ cruel] is likely to form. By contrast, if a person is often told, "That was really kind of you" and "What a sweet thing to do," a relation such as [what I do ≈ kind ≈ sweet] may form. Interestingly, the research suggests that different relations may become active in different contextual situations, which may explain in part why someone is often a "different person" in one setting than in another and why personality is highly situation specific (Mischel, 1968, 1986).

ACCEPTANCE AND COMMITMENT

The value of acceptance has long been recognized. The Serenity Prayer ("Grant me the serenity to accept the things I can't change, the courage to change those I can, and the wisdom to know the difference"), common in substance abuse work, is a familiar example. In recent years, however, the specific usefulness of acceptance-based approaches in professional treatment and consultation has received significant attention (Hayes, Jacobson, Follette, & Dougher, 1994). For example, in couples work, although active procedures such as contracting are valuable, behaviorists have increasingly noted that many stable, overlearned behavior patterns may be difficult to change. In some cases in which such patterns are not abusive or highly disruptive, the most effective approach may be for spouses to learn to accept them, while emphasizing only a few key areas for change (Koerner, Jacobson, & Christensen, 1994).

In work with individual clients, the worker and client must first identify what situations should and what situations should not be accepted by the client. Clearly, it would be a mistake, and often unethical, to encourage clients to accept everything (for example, an abusive relationship). There are some categories of circumstances that one is best off to ultimately accept (although doing so may involve a process; see below); some that one does best to accept for now, with expectation of eventual change; and others that one can often change in the moment. These categories are spelled out in Figure 4-4.

Physical reality and history cannot be changed and are ultimately best accepted. If a client is disturbed by memories of past events, a process of exposure (see below) may be useful in attenuating accompanying emotions, and sometimes the client can take active steps to change the current outcomes of the events. That the events occurred, however, is best accepted. The current feelings associated with such memories should be accepted for now (Freud recognized the negative effects of repression and denial), although one may take active steps now that may later lead to emotional changes.

Reasons always exist for why one feels the way one does. From a behavioral perspective, emotions are states of the body and are the result of current conditions (both in the outside environment as well as within) and learning history. Telling someone, "Don't be sad," therefore, is under most conditions unlikely to be an effective intervention. ACT (Hayes & Wilson, 1994) is a recently developed behavioral approach for addressing situations in which emotional states seem to paralyze the client and prevent him or her from

Domains in which acceptance is useful
- Events and memories from one's own and others' histories
- One's own past acts
- Actions of others over which one has no influence, or which have no genuinely aversive impact on oneself or others
- The physical world

Domains in which current acceptance, with commitment to act to achieve change, can be useful
- One's own emotions (which are responsive to current life events and conditions)
- Others' unpleasant emotional experiences
- Firmly held beliefs of others
- Behavior of others over which one has potential influence, and which has a genuinely aversive impact on one's own or others' lives

Domains in which an emphasis on change is useful
- Self-talk and beliefs that prove inconsistent with events
- One's own undesirable overt behavior
- Aversive situations, except those that are inherently unchangeable

Figure 4-4. Domains in which acceptance, acceptance with commitment to change, and change strategies may be useful in enhancing quality of life.

taking necessary actions. Although ACT is a complex approach that includes a number of useful techniques, a simple beginning with broad applicability to clinical social work will be sketched here.

The central core of ACT is a change in verbal behavior. Rather than saying to oneself (or others), "I want to take that step, *but* I am too anxious (or depressed or angry or whatever) to do so," one instead learns to say, "I want to take that step, *and* I am very anxious about it." The change is, at first glance, small but potentially profound. The first statement suggests that one must first change the way one feels and then take steps toward achieving one's goals. The second statement suggests that a person can often determine what he or she wants to do, acknowledge (not deny) the related feeling (because emotions are natural responses to current conditions and life experience), but still commit to taking the steps necessary to reach one's goals. Too simple? Yes and no; yes, because many of the other interventive strategies presented here also may be needed for success, and no, because clinical experience suggests that this critical change can be extremely powerful. Rather than fighting the feeling, one can observe oneself having the feeling but still act.

Simply observing oneself having feelings and recognizing—and accepting—that those feelings are the natural outcome of current conditions and

Clinical Practice with Individuals

one's experiences also can be freeing. Clients often condemn themselves for having feelings that they have been told are negative (anxiety, sadness, anger) and, as a result, try to fight off these natural reactions and then experience worse feelings because they are having the original feeling. Thinking of emotions as natural under the circumstances, on the other hand, lets a person accept the feelings and take steps that in the long run will lead to relief. In the short run, fighting emotions typically only makes them worse; as Hayes and Wilson (1994) suggested, if you cannot accept the feeling for now, you will be stuck with it, but if you can, you can change your world so you will not have that feeling later. Highly verbal clients often quickly generalize this concept to new situations they face, whereas those with less complex verbal repertoires may require a good deal of assistance from the social worker to accept their feelings in specific situations.

One client of mine was unhappy that he was sensitive to (and badly wanted) others' approval. He was a successful professional but wanted to "kill the monster" that hungered for admiration from others. Once he saw this desire as a natural response emerging from his life experience, he immediately understood that he could not "kill" his monster but had to tame it. It was a part of himself that he had no choice but to accept, but he need not take it too seriously. He also was able to generalize this new approach to other undesirable emotions and quickly learned to observe and accept feelings and then to decide whether he wished to respond to them in his ordinary manner.

By contrast, a current client of mine, also very bright but somewhat incapacitated by depression, is able to agree that in specific situations her demoralization is natural given her intense social isolation but so far needs continuing help to plan, commit to, and execute specific tasks toward her goals. She still finds it difficult to generalize normalization and acceptance of emotions to novel situations, although she can do it with help. Many clients, particularly those who suffer from depression or have limited verbal repertoires, may require such guidance.

EXPOSURE

Clients often see social workers or other professionals because they want to change unpleasant emotional states such as anxiety or anger. One approach, which is often effective in these cases, is to work with the client to change related self-talk. In some cases this change may be adequate in itself, but often the best results come from combining this work with exposure. Anxiety is a good example. Sometimes the origins of an anxiety problem are clear, as in the case of a client who often feels anxious in enclosed spaces such as elevators (claustrophobic) and remembers being frightened when locked in a closet by an older brother when growing up. In other cases, the origin of the anxiety may be obscure, as for a client who engages in compulsive rituals that may once have served to distract from other sources of known or unknown stress (abuse, for example) but now have taken on a life of their own. Such clients often feel anxious if they do not engage in the rituals. There is a strong respondent (classical conditioning) component in such problems.

The central task in such cases is to expose oneself to the anxiety-provoking situation without experiencing negative consequences. There are several variations for doing so, but they all share this common core. Changing self-talk is often useful as part of this program; for example, many people experiencing panic attacks believe that they are having a heart attack, are unable to get enough oxygen to survive, or in some other way are at imminent risk of death or other severe consequence. For a generally healthy person this is not true, and learning that fact and reminding oneself of it during the attack is often enough to attenuate and sometimes to end the attack. Exposure to stimuli similar to attacks (which can be brought about by hyperventilating or other procedures) combined with changing self-talk is usually an effective package (Craske & Barlow, 1993).

Exposure can be carried out in many ways. A person who becomes anxious in stores can either spend a good deal of time in stores (often with a supportive person such as the social worker present at first) all at once (*flooding*) or can work his or her way up to that in small manageable steps. Either can work; flooding is usually faster, but graduated exposure is generally considerably less aversive. In graduated exposure, a plan is developed for experiencing the feared situation in a mild way initially and then proceeding gradually through more difficult steps until the most difficult can be tolerated. A person who becomes panicky in stores might begin by parking outside the store until that can be tolerated, then move to standing outside the door of the store for a while. In the next exposure session, he or she might practice those steps again, then simply walk into and back out of the store, and so forth.

Several types of supports can be useful in this process, including practicing new self-talk during exposure, performing relaxation exercises, or being accompanied by a trusting person. Coping self-talk can be cued by a small card the client carries with him or her during the process. Relaxation was once usually paired with exposure in a procedure called *systematic desensitization*; research indicated that the relaxation component was not necessary for effectiveness, but relaxation exercises (see chapter 5) may help some clients to take the subjective risks involved in exposure. If a trusted person accompanies the client during early stages of exposure, that person's presence should usually be faded gradually (standing farther away, standing outside the building, waiting in the car, waiting by a phone, and so forth) in a planned way to make the transition as easy as possible. If any stage in a graduated exposure program proves too anxiety provoking, it is usually best to go back and practice an easier stage further before again attempting the more difficult step.

Some professionals once believed that using such behavioral techniques for anxiety disorders would result in "symptom substitution," in which the client would just start experiencing a new problem, because exposure might not get at the hypothesized roots of the problem. Symptom substitution has never been demonstrated in years of research, however, and appears to be a myth. At the same time, if a person's anxiety-related symptom has a current function, such as distracting him and his partner from a couple's problem, and if the distracting symptom is removed, the real problem that has been avoided may then become obvious and need to be addressed. Note, however, that this is a different phenomenon than symptom substitution.

An approach related to exposure is *inoculation*. This procedure involves extensive skills training and will therefore be addressed in the next chapter. In that chapter, I outline educational strategies that can be useful for clients by either teaching them new skills needed to obtain adequate satisfaction in their current social and contextual situation or the skills needed to access alternative networks and sources of reinforcers. I place particular emphasis in that discussion on self-monitoring and self-management skills, which are often experienced by clients as particularly empowering strategies.

REFERENCES

Beck, A. T., Freeman, A., & Associates. (1990). *Cognitive therapy of personality disorders.* New York: Guilford Press.

Beck, A. T., Rush, A. J., Shaw, B. F., & Emery, G. (1978). *Cognitive therapy of depression.* New York: Guilford Press.

Craske, M. G., & Barlow, D. H. (1993). Panic disorder and agoraphobia. In D. H. Barlow (Ed.), *Clinical handbook of psychological disorders* (pp. 1–47). New York: Guilford Press.

Dougher, M. J., & Hackbert, L. (1994). A behavior-analytic account of depression and a case report using acceptance-based procedures. *Behavior Analyst, 17,* 321–334.

Ellis, A., & Whitely, J. M. (1979). *Theoretical and empirical foundations of rational-emotive therapy.* Monterey, CA: Brooks/Cole.

Goldfried, M. R., & Davison, G. C. (1976). *Clinical behavior therapy.* New York: Holt, Rinehart & Winston.

Hayes, S. C., Jacobson, N. S., Follette, V. M., & Dougher, M. J. (Eds.). (1994). *Acceptance and change: Content and context in psychotherapy.* Reno, NV: Context Press.

Hayes, S. C., & Wilson, K. G. (1994). Acceptance and commitment therapy: Altering the verbal support for experiential avoidance. *Behavior Analyst, 17,* 289–303.

Hayes, S. C., Zettle, R. D., & Rosenfarb, I. (1989). Rule-following. In S. C. Hayes (Ed.), *Rule-governed behavior: Cognition, contingencies, and instructional control* (pp. 191–220). New York: Plenum Press.

Koerner, K., Jacobson, N. S., & Christensen, A. (1994). Emotional acceptance in integrative behavioral couple therapy. In S. C. Hayes, N. S. Jacobson, V. M. Follette, & M. J. Dougher (Eds.), *Acceptance and change: Content and context in psychotherapy* (pp. 109–118). Reno, NV: Context Press.

Kohlenberg, R. J., & Tsai, M. (1991). *Functional analytic psychotherapy: Creating intense and curative therapeutic relationships.* New York: Plenum Press.

Mischel, W. (1968). *Personality and assessment.* New York: John Wiley & Sons.

Mischel, W. (1986). *Introduction to personality: A new look* (4th ed.). New York: Holt, Rinehart & Winston.

Reid, W. J. (1985). *Family problem solving.* New York: Columbia University Press.

Yankura, J., & Dryden, W. (1990). *Doing RET: Albert Ellis in action.* New York: Springer.

CHAPTER FIVE

INTERVENTIVE STRATEGIES: SKILLS TRAINING

S kills training has long been associated with behavioral approaches to practice because many clients have not learned effective repertoires for achieving an adequate fit with their environments or do not use existing repertoires on appropriate occasions. (Work with private events is a special case of skills training.) Examples of areas in which this educational strategy may be valuable include social skills training (for example, assertion training), teaching parenting skills, relaxation training, and stress inoculation. Training may focus on specific skills such as conversation openers as well as subtle repertoires (for example, learning to talk about what is right rather than what is wrong with one's life).

Techniques used in skills training, regardless of the content, commonly include a description of the desired behaviors, discussion of the advantages of learning new skills (to increase motivation), modeling (in which the social worker or someone else demonstrates the skill), rehearsal (practicing, often in a role-played situation), and explicit reinforcement and feedback. The relative mix among these depends on the skills to be learned. In parent training, for example, the components of giving a small child clear directions are well known and can be taught in a straightforward manner. Carrying on an interesting conversation in social situations, by contrast, is a complex, multidimensional repertoire. Some aspects of the latter are clear; for example, asking questions about the other person's interests. However, other dimensions, including body position, distance, tone of voice, and other subtle actions cannot universally be captured by a few simple rules. One approach to such situations is to give the client global feedback about the relative effectiveness of multiple trials, along with specific guidance where possible. Some research suggests that this contingency-shaped approach to social skills training may be more effective than the rule-governed alternative (Hayes, Zettle, & Rosenfarb, 1989).

Additional discussion of social skills training, which is broadly useful for relationship issues and constructing social repertoires that are likely to be effective under various conditions, is found in chapter 8. This chapter outlines four other classes of skills with broad applicability to many clinical situations: self-monitoring, self-management, relaxation, and inoculation.

SELF-MONITORING

Self-monitoring is a simple and effective intervention strategy. In self-monitoring, clients themselves collect data regarding behavior or experiences. For example, clients who are demoralized often will report that they are always unhappy, and it may be difficult to determine exactly what is happening in their lives. If clients have reasonably strong related repertoires (for example, literacy and recordkeeping), they may be able to keep a record such as that shown in Figure 2-6 (p. 37). The 23-year-old woman who collected those data was asked to note what she was doing during all waking hours and her level of satisfaction on roughly an hour-by-hour basis. This kind of record often provides significant information regarding the conditions and events that a client finds particularly reinforcing or aversive and patterns linking emotional experiences with environmental factors, which can be useful in deciding on the types of active experiments to try. Many clients find such records both easy to keep and helpful for understanding how their experiences relate to environmental factors.

However, self-monitoring can do more; it can help a client gain a sense of control over his or her life and therefore is an important tool for empowerment (Kopp, 1993). It is often useful to set a goal (such as spending more time with friends, beginning an exercise regimen, or praising your child more often), but actually seeing the progress can make a substantial difference, especially if you are sharing the data with someone else, such as the social worker, who can provide additional reinforcement. At this point self-monitoring is more than an assessment tool; it is an active intervention, in which reactivity to the procedure is not only acceptable, but desirable. It may seem that setting the goal and estimating how well you have done would be adequate, but it is not nearly as powerful as actual monitoring, even though the latter may feel artificial at first. In many areas it is not too strong to say that if records are not kept, lasting change will not occur.

Many types of data can be collected through self-monitoring. It is possible to track the frequency of specifically targeted behaviors, including such things as telephone calls made to look for jobs, hours spent doing homework, or intentionally providing verbal reinforcement for positive actions of an intimate partner or supervisee. It is also possible to keep track of private events, such as the number of times (and how badly) one craves cigarettes or level of tension, anger, or pleasure experienced over time. One important consideration is to provide the client with ways to make monitoring as simple and accurate as possible. Simple tools, such as a plastic golf counter carried in a pocket, a piece of paper and pencil in a cigarette pack, a chart kept on the refrigerator door, or a small card with a self-anchored scale printed on it, are extremely useful, and it is a good idea to keep a supply of such things in a drawer for cases in which they may be needed. Clients can be asked to develop their own charts; for those who can, doing this provides an additional level of personal control. Many clients, however, need the clinician to provide the tools. (People who find self-monitoring valuable may want to invest in wristwatches with built-in lap counters, which can be used to keep track of many different types of data over time.)

Social workers should try self-monitoring themselves to experience both the benefits and the challenges involved (most will find a need for a commitment to show the data to someone else if they want to be consistent). Although self-monitoring as a stand-alone technique is useful, its power can be leveraged when it is incorporated as one component of a self-management program.

SELF-MANAGEMENT

Self-management strategies have been used by people interested in improving their health status in ways that are more effective than "resolutions," including maintaining exercise programs, proper nutrition, and smoking cessation. Clearly, this approach is broadly applicable in making personal changes and can be helpful in supporting the sorts of experiments with life discussed in earlier chapters.

Data from an exercise self-management program are shown in Figure 5-1. During the baseline period, in a typical pattern for unassisted resolutions, the frequency of exercise began at a reasonably high but inconsistent level but then fairly quickly dropped off. Once the self-management program was

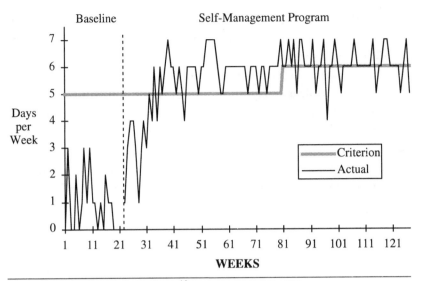

Figure 5-1. Data from an exercise self-management program.

initiated, however, the rate became quite consistent and was maintained for the subsequent two years. An effective self-management plan has four critical steps, none of which can safely be omitted. The first step is to identify a goal; this may be improved health, an improved relationship, or finding a job. Establishing the goal typically occurs during the assessment process, when the client determines, with the worker's assistance, how he or she wants his or her life to be different. The goal should be genuinely important to the client and not something that someone else wants the client to do or consistency in self-management is unlikely. It is sometimes useful to spend time in motivational interviewing (Miller & Rollnick, 1991), in which the worker discusses with the client the reasons for the goal and the long-term advantages of pursuing it and disadvantages of not pursuing it.

Once the goal is clearly defined, the client–worker team should pinpoint the actions that they believe will lead to reaching the goal. For example, if the client wants to improve or maintain health, as in the example in Figure 5-1, exercise is usually an important component. (Note that exercise is often a critical ingredient in managing many emotional and mood issues as well but is typically among the most difficult steps for a client to pursue when not feeling "strong.") The man whose data are shown in Figure 5-1 decided that he should engage in any of several types of exercise (primarily walking for an

Clinical Practice with Individuals

hour a day but with other acceptable alternatives) at least six days per week. This level of precision is essential; one must pinpoint the precise behavior required and its targeted frequency. Some of these objectives are best established on a daily basis; with others, a weekly cumulative total may be more workable. Clients nearly always try to establish initial pinpoints that are too difficult; the worker should strongly advise setting a relatively easy objective in the beginning (which the client is free to exceed). More challenging objectives can then be set as easier ones are met.

The third step is to establish a plan for monitoring the pinpointed behavior and tracking it in a reliable way. For example, most people are not good at remembering how many times in the past week they exercised, and some of the benefits of self-monitoring, including looking at one's performance regularly, also are lost in retrospective reconstruction of data. A chart or graph kept in a standard and accessible place is usually best; for many people this means on the refrigerator door, but it can also be on an office wall, in a wallet, or wherever it is most available when the data should be entered, depending on the person and the desired action.

Up to this point, the steps in self-management are essentially those of self-monitoring. What more might be needed? The pinpointed objectives established (and being monitored) are behavioral, of course. Remember that the primary determinants of behavior are consequences. Effective self-management often requires careful examination and usually planning around consequences. Many people think that, by making a commitment to themselves, they will consistently act according to their plan. In cases in which the repertoires are easy for the person to emit and have major immediate automatic payoffs, this may be true. In most cases of self-management, however, relying on self-discipline in this way proves to be self-deception. If the desired changes were easy to make, the client would usually have made them long ago.

Natural contingencies are often inadequate to establish and maintain many valued actions because they require a long series of small cumulative actions to achieve and because the outcome often remains uncertain. For example, one must read many pages to finish a degree; often it is unknown which material will be on the test. Under those circumstances, going to a movie or even doing the dishes may be more likely than studying. Similarly, depressed clients must consistently and often leave the house and socialize with other people; this process requires considerable effort and produces no immediate improvement in feelings. It is easy to understand why a person in that situation may put off taking action.

Consequences can be addressed several ways in self-management. First, it is important to examine how the existing situation may make it difficult for the client to take the steps he or she wants to by punishing the desired action; by providing inadequate, delayed, or uncertain reinforcers for the desired action; or by reinforcing less desirable alternatives. In some cases, these potential situational obstacles can be overcome, but it is always important to recognize them. Second, behavior sometimes responds to monitoring by oneself alone, but most things that are difficult require that commitments be made and data be shared regularly (at least weekly) with someone else. In part, this sharing of data may involve avoidance of a mild aversive situation (for example, potential embarrassment), but ideally the person assisting in monitoring also can provide recognition and appreciation for positive steps that have been taken (even if adherence to the plan is less than perfect, although one must be cautious not to reinforce excellent "excuse-giving"). The social worker is usually a good choice as a performance monitor in the beginning; often it may be useful to shift this role to someone in the client's natural environment as quickly as possible.

Finally, small but immediate consequences are often useful for keeping a self-management program on track. Although people sometimes feel that these steps are trivial or silly, they seem to work well and should not be discounted. If a self-management program is not working, more attention to these small steps is important. Two basic approaches exist to consequation: arranging reinforcers and using mild, self-administered penalties. Reinforcers may be tangible (for example, for every day I exercise this week, I can spend an additional $2 when I go shopping on Saturday on something I usually would not buy) or may involve activities (if I meet my goal of praising my child 50 times this week, I can watch a favorite television show next week).

Although reinforcers are usually the best way to change behavior, many people have found that small, self-imposed penalties that are easy to avoid are not very aversive and are a quick and easy way to ensure compliance with their plan (which later results in substantial reinforcement). For example, I generally have about a dozen self-management programs in place at any time. Although I use reinforcers for some particularly challenging objectives on occasion, small fines (say $1 per day for each missed objective, paid to an organization) for missing my objectives work well, in large part as reminders of the pinpointed behaviors. However, most important consequences are social; I report my progress once a week to a colleague who does the same with me. Before establishing this reporting system, consistent, stable progress was never achieved. For clients, a similar reporting and monitoring arrangement is usually crucial.

The four critical steps in self-management, then, are to (1) establish the goal, (2) pinpoint specific steps toward the goal, (3) develop and implement a monitoring plan, and (4) ensure adequate reinforcers or other consequences are in place to support the pinpointed behaviors. Examples of self-management strategies are found in many of the subsequent chapters. Note that self-management as a strategy is applicable not only to health-related behaviors or those involved in achieving work or academic goals. Self-management strategies also have broad clinical use for problems such as substance abuse, depression, and relationship issues. Self-management is ultimately about taking control of the contingencies that shape one's behavior; this is why it is an empowering strategy.

RELAXATION

One valuable skill, often included in self-management programs, is relaxation exercises. Relaxation skills are seldom an adequate interventive strategy on their own but are often useful as one component in clinical consultation. Learning how to relax (to modify visceral processes) can be helpful as a way of providing immediate relief for anxious clients who may find it difficult to concentrate or communicate in sessions as well as for application in life situations in which excessive tension or anxiety interferes with the client's ability to function.

Relaxation skills can be learned and improved through practice (like other skills such as playing sports or driving a car). It is important to let clients know that improvement is likely to be gradual and that in the beginning they may find it difficult to apply these repertoires effectively in challenging situations. Many clients also find that the immediate relief they experience when practicing these techniques with the social worker provides a sense of hope for change. It is usually best for the client to practice first with the worker because many clients will place demands for immediate perfection on themselves if they begin in private and some may become more anxious if they notice physiological changes occurring during the process. If the latter occurs, a bit of reassurance that this means the technique is beginning to work is usually adequate; if not, the worker may want to suggest a technique from a different class of relaxation exercises. In a very few cases, difficulties experienced by the client may be reflections of resistance, in which case the issues involved may need to be explored (see chapter 2).

Relaxation skills can be used in two primary ways that can contribute to each other. One way is to develop a regular regimen of relaxation (or variations, including meditation; see below) that may be useful in reducing the overall level of stress experienced in daily life. Ten to 20 minutes once or twice per day is a reasonable target. Significant mental and physical health benefits appear to be associated with this sort of regimen (Benson, 1975); this association may explain why many cultural traditions around the world include some form of regular meditation or physiologically based alternative. Many people find that incorporating a relaxation component into their self-management plans (see previous section) is useful because it is difficult to maintain this kind of program through sheer willpower.

A second way to use relaxation skills is to cope with high-stress situations at the moment they are occurring. To be effective in this way the skills must be well learned in advance (an inoculation program, discussed in the next section, is a useful way to achieve fluency). Simple and often brief relaxation techniques are called for in these circumstances. Some useful ones include taking three deep, increasingly slow breaths (ideally while covertly verbalizing a word that has been practiced and has become associated with relaxation; see below). Changing stimulus conditions—for example, by looking out a window or going to another room—is often useful while doing this. Two other useful approaches include making a fist (without threatening anyone) then gradually relaxing the hand (tension/relaxation) or letting go of tension in a particular body part, such as the shoulders, that the client has identified as consistently tight under tense circumstances (letting go). Many variations of these techniques can be adapted individually by the client and worker.

Each of the following is a brief version of one of the common types of relaxation techniques (although extensive overlap occurs):

- breathing (for example, the relaxation response, rhythmic breathing)
- muscle relaxation (for example, tension/relaxation or letting go)
- visualization (for example, in imagination or reality)
- interrupting excessive self-talk

Clinical Practice with Individuals

- incorporating movement or body positioning (for example, tai chi or yoga).

In addition, many people find that they can achieve similar benefits through regular vigorous exercise or the practice of some form of martial arts. Techniques such as yoga generally require considerable instruction to learn, but there are simple and highly effective versions of the other types available. An example of each is presented here.

The Relaxation Response

Herbert Benson of Harvard University developed a simple technique to elicit what he called the *relaxation response*, a physiological pattern of deep relaxation that research suggests can be obtained through a wide variety of relaxation and meditation approaches (Benson, 1975). The simple steps recommended by Benson are as follows:
- Take a comfortable position in a quiet environment.
- Close your eyes, adopt a passive attitude, and become aware of your breathing.
- Breathe very slowly, and each time you exhale, repeat a word (Benson recommended the word "one," but any word that is meaningful to the client will work, for example, "relax," "peace," or "yes").
- Continue this process for 10 to 20 minutes. When distractions occur, which they will, passively set them aside. *It is not important to avoid distractions, only not to take them seriously.*

This technique is easy to teach to clients. It is helpful to provide the client with written, step-by-step instructions, to plan together what time of day to practice the technique (it should be done almost every day), and to work up a self-monitoring/self-management plan. Because of its simplicity, it is an excellent choice as a first relaxation technique to offer to clients. (In many cases the clinician and client may want to experiment with several techniques before deciding which to rely on.)

Tension/Relaxation

A relaxation technique based on tensing then relaxing various muscle groups called *progressive muscle relaxation* has proved useful in clinical work for decades (Jacobson, 1929). This technique is especially effective with clients who are particularly aware of the physiological sensations they experience when they are tense. The social worker should first ask whether the client has any physical problems that might be bothered by tensing and relaxing muscles; those areas of the body should be avoided during the exercise. Begin by asking the client to settle back in a comfortable position and close his or her eyes. Then provide instructions roughly like the following, in a slow and calming voice, using long pauses:

> Now just settle back, close your eyes and relax . . . breathe slowly and evenly . . . even a bit slower . . . good. . . . Now turn your attention to your right hand . . . make a fist, tensing your hand about halfway, and hold the tension . . . just notice the tension in your hand . . . hold it . . . and now slowly relax it . . . just let go . . . further and further . . . until your hand feels very, very relaxed . . . now turn your attention to your left hand.

The same basic instructions are given for each part of the body in succession, each time emphasizing tensing, holding the tension, then letting go. Minor variations and elaborations can be used throughout such as, "notice how different the relaxation feels from the tension you felt before" and "even though your shoulders now feel very relaxed, see if you can let go even a bit further." Remind the client periodically that it is necessary to tense only about halfway and to continue to breathe slowly and evenly. Although the order of moving through the body can vary, the following order works well (specific guidance for several body parts as noted here can be helpful):

- hands
- lower arms (making a fist but also tensing up to the elbow)
- biceps and upper arms (have the client raise his or her hands into fists near the face during the tensing phase)
- feet (curling toes tightly)
- calves (pressing down on the floor with feet)
- thighs
- buttocks
- lower back (arching back—be certain the client has no history of back problems)
- stomach/diaphragm area (suck in)
- chest (lift and hold)
- shoulders (lift toward ears and hold)
- front of neck (bury chin in chest)
- back of neck (arch backwards)
- face (grimace, tensing all facial muscles).

In ending the exercise, the worker can have the client sit quietly for one or two minutes and then say, "Now, I'm going to count backwards from three to one. When I reach one, you will be wide awake but still very relaxed . . . three . . . two . . . waking up . . . one. Wide awake. You can open your eyes and stretch a bit now." (Occasionally someone falls asleep during this exercise. When that happens, the clinician can simply wake the client.) It is possible to tape these instructions while taking the client through the technique for later use at home. Although I am aware of no data on this, my clinical experience suggests that a self-monitoring plan is essential if the client wants to use such a tape regularly; otherwise, it is too easy to procrastinate.

Visualization

Many visualization techniques have been used to achieve deep states of relaxation, from imagining a flower slowly blossoming to imaging events occurring in the body (Van Over, 1978). One common visualization exercise that I have used extensively is outlined in Figure 5-2 (readers should use their own geographic settings and landmarks).

When using this exercise, the idea is not only to become very relaxed but also to imagine oneself becoming more and more distant from the small concerns of daily life. Relaxation techniques can be integrated with acceptance and commitment techniques to achieve a coherent package in which oneself, one's actions and emotions, and life events are accepted as naturally connected phenomena.

Interrupting Negative Self-Talk or Imaging

Many clients worry about the future or focus excessively on negative events from the past, either in the form of self-talk or remembering scenes (covert observation). One of the functions of any relaxation technique is to interrupt these patterns and provide a period of relief. Additional techniques involve essentially attending to alternative words or images. For example, collections of "Zen art," images that can be used as the focus of meditation exercises, are available (Holmes & Horioka, 1973). One example is shown in Figure 5-3.

The client can begin a 10- to 20-minute period of relaxation by first concentrating on and slowing his or her breathing, then focusing on such an image, and returning to it whenever distractions intrude. Some clients may prefer to move slowly, gently, and passively through several such images during one relaxation period. For other clients, or at other times, verbal tools

[Insert pauses throughout; aim for a slow, easy pace and a relaxing tone and quality of voice.]

Just settle back into your chair . . . find a comfortable position, and close your eyes . . .

Now imagine that your body is becoming more relaxed, and also lighter . . . bit by bit, lighter and lighter . . .

And imagine that as your body becomes lighter, it begins to be able to float just above the chair . . . you are still anchored to the chair somehow, but your body can gently drift upward, toward the ceiling . . .

And you can float right through the ceiling, through the upper stories of this building, and very gently, right through the roof . . . you feel quite safe, you can still see the chair and could return at any time, but you continue to float . . . lighter and lighter . . .

As you rise higher, you can see the entire block . . . you can see Broadway, you notice all the activity there, but somehow it doesn't seem so important from this vantage point . . . you just keep gently rising, higher and higher . . .

Now you can see the Hudson, and now the East River . . . and all of Manhattan Island . . . gently continuing to float upward . . .

Now you can see Long Island, and the Atlantic . . . higher and higher . . .

And now, all of North America . . . you still feel connected to your physical body here in this room, but your floating self can see the globe, and gazing out, look into the vastness of space . . .

And you just remain there for a few minutes, gently floating, looking down on the earth, and recognizing that many of the things that seemed so important down there really aren't . . . just gently letting go of any tension and worries . . . very peaceful . . . notice how relaxed you are now . . .

Now you can very gently begin to return, to drift downward very slowly, moving closer to the earth . . . gradually Manhattan comes back into view . . .

And as you slowly return, you begin to make out details of New York City . . . Broadway . . . you can see the cars . . . the people . . . and very gently, you settle back toward this building . . .

Returning, floating down, coming back into this room . . . and into your chair . . . still very relaxed and peaceful . . .

Now, I am going to count backwards from three to one. With each number, you will feel more alert and awake, but still very relaxed . . . three . . . waking up . . . two . . . becoming more alert . . . one . . . wide awake, very peaceful . . . you can open your eyes when you are ready . . .

Figure 5-2. A visualization exercise for inducing deep relaxation.

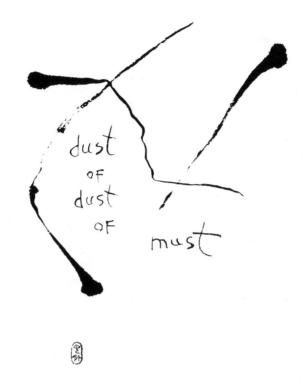

dust
OF
dust
OF
must

Figure 5-3. A zen telegram. Reprinted with permission from Reps, P. (1959). *zen telegrams.* Boston: Charles E. Tuttle, p. 73.

may be used instead of graphics. Poetry or haiku read in a meditative and perhaps a repetitive way can help facilitate reaching a relaxed state, particularly if combined with breathing exercises.

The material presented here is only a partial summary of the wide range of meditation and relaxation strategies. Interestingly, it may not make much difference which strategies are selected, because it appears that all such techniques produce roughly the same kinds of physiological changes (Benson, 1975). Many people find that it is helpful to know several techniques from which they may select based on what feels right at a particular time. One man I know uses breathing exercises much of the time, but when he is particularly distracted or experiencing especially high levels of stress, finds himself too distracted when doing breathing exercises and turns to Zen art. No matter which techniques are selected, make clear to the client that distractions happen. At times the client may feel distracted much of the time during nearly the entire relaxation period, but if he or she accepts the distractions passively and returns to the focus, the expected benefits will still be achieved. Relaxation and self-talk techniques are also key components of inoculation strategies.

INOCULATION

Over the past two decades, inoculation techniques have been demonstrated to be effective for a range of clinical problems, including the management of stress (stress inoculation training) and pain and anger control (see, for example, Davidson, 1976; Goldstein & Keller, 1987). A closely related technique, self-instructional training, emphasizes the self-talk aspects of coping with aversive emotions and other problematic physical states. The core concept of the technique is to rehearse skills that can be used in difficult situations until they become natural and almost automatic. The process is similar across clinical problems; the example of anger management will be presented here. As can be seen in Figure 5-4, there are three phases in a potentially anger-provoking situation.

Clients often know in advance when a situation may be emotionally challenging, and it is valuable to take time to prepare for the provocative situation. As shown in Figure 5-4, useful strategies for this stage include the use of relaxing, coping self-talk; the use of relaxation techniques so one enters the situation in the best possible physiological state; and planning to take steps that may attenuate the problems (for example, arranging to have a third party present or planning to restate the other person's position). During the provocation itself, coping self-talk is again useful, as are emergency relaxation techniques and simple listening and distracting skills. (Some people find it useful to deal with the initial moment of provocation and the continuing conflict process as separate stages.) Finally, after the provocation, self-talk and relaxation techniques for minimizing leftover stress can be useful; perhaps the most valuable skill at this point is self-reinforcement, giving oneself recognition for using the rehearsed skills in the provocative situation (even if not perfectly).

Phase 1: Examples of skills to use in preparing for the provocation:
a) Examples of coping self-talk:
   - "I am strong, I know how to deal with this."
   - "I have the skills I need."
   - "I'm not going to take this too seriously."
   - "I can stay cool."
   - "This is how I plan to handle this situation . . . ."
b) Physiological:
   - Breathing exercises
   - Muscle relaxation exercises
c) Covert rehearsal of the coming provocation, visualizing:
   - Staying calm in the face of it
   - Calmly restating the other's position
   - Acting nonprovokingly
d) Taking steps to attenuate the conflict:
   - Have a third party present
   - Prepare possible compromises or solutions

Phase 2: Examples of skills to use during the provocation:
a) Examples of coping self-talk:
   - "Stay cool."
   - "We both deserve respect."
   - "Don't take it seriously."
   - "I'm in control. I can be strong in the face of this."
   - "This isn't so bad; I can handle it."
   - "He is very unhappy, it's too bad."
   - "We can find a solution to this."
   - "I won't let him control my emotions."
b) Physiological:
   - Focus on relaxing high-tension points (shoulders, hands).
   - Take several deep breaths, hold them, and let them out slowly.
c) Verbal:
   - Paraphrase what the other says.
   - State the other's interests.
   - Suggest solutions.
   - Inject humor when appropriate.
   - Remain nonprovoking.

Phase 3: Examples of skills to use after the provocative situation:
a) Self-talk:
   - "I handled that pretty well"
   - "The part I handled best was when I . . ."
   - "It wasn't perfect, but it was real progress for me"
   - "The next time, I could . . ."
b) Covert or overt rehearsal of the situation to explore other ways to handle similar situations in the future
c) Relaxation skills to reduce arousal.

Figure 5-4. Skills to be rehearsed for dealing with the three phases of a potentially anger-provoking situation.

In anger inoculation training, the first step is educational; the worker begins by presenting the rationale and overall plan to the client. The client and worker then work together to decide on specific skills for each stage, including verbal and physiological tactics, that seem like the best fit for the client (experimentation may be required). Those skills chosen should be few in number so the client can remember them, but there should be several for each stage so the client feels as if he or she has an adequate repertoire in case one tactic does not work. Perhaps the most crucial stage of the training is rehearsing the use of the skills in simulated situations. These are role-played, beginning with mildly challenging conflicts and then progressing to more difficult ones in which the worker may take the role of a significant other who "gets in the client's face" and says hurtful things in a loud and angry voice. The more practice the client has in the session and in real-life situations, the better he or she is likely to become at coping, because like any skills, these require practice.

Inoculation training is usually done in a structured way, with the stages and tactics for each situation carefully planned, written out, and practiced. Assignments to use the skills outside the session in the client's life-space are important both to encourage generalization and to provide more extensive practice. Most of the strategies and skills discussed throughout this chapter will be most useful to the client if they are practiced regularly in the client's daily life. Although the clinical session is useful as a forum for teaching, problem solving, and planning, with most clients, some form of home assignment should routinely be used between sessions. Whenever possible, it is valuable to conduct sessions in the client's world rather than the worker's. A client practicing relaxation skills at his or her own office or parenting skills in his or her own home with his or her own child is more likely to continue to use those skills, because the stimulus conditions remain largely the same. Although home sessions are time-consuming and involve many challenges in terms of ensuring structure and negotiating to prevent interruptions, they are among the clinician's most powerful tools and should be used whenever possible. Home sessions greatly simplify generalization and maintenance, as discussed in chapter 6.

REFERENCES

Benson, H. (1975). *The relaxation response.* New York: Avon Books.

Davidson, P. O. (Ed.). (1976). *The behavioral management of anxiety, depression and pain.* New York: Brunner/Mazel.

Goldstein, A. P., & Keller, H. (1987). *Aggressive behavior: Assessment and intervention.* New York: Pergamon Press.

Hayes, S. C., Zettle, R. D., & Rosenfarb, I. (1989). Rule-following. In S. C. Hayes (Ed.), *Rule-governed behavior: Cognition, contingencies, and instructional control* (pp. 191–220). New York: Plenum Press.

Holmes, S. W., & Horioka, C. (1973). *Zen art for meditation.* Boston: Charles E. Tuttle.

Jacobson, E. (1929). *Progressive relaxation.* Chicago: University of Chicago Press.

Kopp, J. (1993). Self-observation: An empowerment strategy in assessment. In J. B. Rauch (Ed.), *Assessment: A sourcebook for social work practice* (pp. 255–268). Milwaukee: Families International.

Miller, W. R., & Rollnick, S. (1991). *Motivational interviewing: Preparing people to change addictive behavior.* New York: Guilford Press.

Reps, P. (1959). *zen telegrams.* Boston: Charles E. Tuttle.

Van Over, R. (1978). *Total meditation.* New York: Collier.

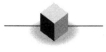

CHAPTER SIX

ESTABLISHING AND MAINTAINING CHANGE IN THE NATURAL ENVIRONMENT

The client's natural environment usually is not like the social worker's office, and just as the perpetual motion machine does not exist, a "perpetual-behavior intervention" does not exist either (Malott, Whaley, & Malott, 1993). Only behavior that results in an adequate level of reinforcement under current conditions will be maintained reliably, so intervention planning must consider how new behaviors will transfer to the client's natural environment and how they will be reinforced there. Many clients who learn an assertive or parenting skill well in the office do not apply it in their natural environments; many clients whose depression lifted became depressed again a few months later. Although there is no easy way to achieve transfer (often called *generalization*) and maintenance of change, there also is nothing mystical about how to go about doing so. The material that follows looks first at transfer of newly learned skills to the natural environment and then at maintenance.

TRANSFER TO THE NATURAL ENVIRONMENT

Intervening directly in the client's life-space eliminates the need to transfer skills to the natural environment. Think about a young child having behavior problems in school; under many circumstances it is relatively easy to resolve such issues behaviorally in the classroom (Ginsburg, 1990) and more difficult to do so through counseling sessions in the office (as always, a careful assessment should be done to ensure that the behavior is not the result of a problem elsewhere). Similarly in clinical practice, two strategies are used to eliminate concern about generalization: (1) to do all or most of the clinical consultation in the client's normal environment or (2) to extensively assign tasks to be done at home or in other natural settings. In addition, a set of procedural variations may help in achieving transfer. Each of these strategies is summarized in the material that follows.

Work in the Client's Natural Environment

Social work has always used the "home visit." Clinical consultation for nearly any issue can often be effectively provided in the home. If a client practices new social skills or new forms of verbal behavior (such as talking about what is positive rather than what is wrong) at home in his or her living room or kitchen, these new skills can to some extent come under the stimulus control of those places and may be more easily evoked there in the future. Self-monitoring charts can be developed and posted in the home during the session. A client can telephone a friend from his or her own room or learn relaxation exercises in the setting (and under the possibly distracting conditions) where he or she is being asked to practice them.

Working in the home also provides richer data for assessment. The clinician can learn a great deal about the natural contingencies present in a client's life by directly observing the street outside, the neighbors, others living in the home, and the physical environment. Some depressed clients may live under dark and deprived conditions, and changes in these conditions may make a meaningful difference. The relationship between worker and client may also develop more naturally and with a less pronounced power differential, and the client may act in a more typical way in the home than in the foreign and often stressful setting of the professional office.

Disadvantages to work in the home also may occur. Social workers should not put themselves at needless risk by entering a home alone where there is a substantial chance of physical attack or other danger. It may be important to select the best time of day to visit. Home visiting may not be as cost-effective as working in the office because of the need for travel or clients who are not at home when the visit is made. Still, clients live where they do, and a worker or agency willing to make the commitment of visiting despite obstacles communicates a strong message of respect and commitment. In some fields of practice, home visiting is mandated, but in most others it is useful.

Home Tasks

In ecobehavioral practice, with nearly every client in every session, a major emphasis is on developing experiments to be tried, data to be collected, or skills to be practiced between sessions in the natural environment. It is in the natural environment that the client is asking and hoping for change—not in the social worker's office. The real test of intervention, therefore, is always change (or maintenance) in the client's life situation. Collaboratively developed home tasks build a clear and crucial bridge between the office and the real world in ways that merely achieving insight into why things are not going as well as one might hope cannot. Home assignments or home tasks are, therefore, routinely used in ecobehavioral (and task-centered; Reid, 1992) practice approaches.

For example, a client's tasks might be to experiment with providing verbal reinforcement to others in the family 20 times in the coming week and to keep track of the times he or she has done so and the results in writing. This kind of assignment is more likely to produce change than simply recognizing that one is not very positive with family members. Another client may take on the task of acting like her assertive sister on the job for two days and then reporting what happened. Experiencing the resulting consequences is far more powerful than imagining them and is often crucial to gradually shaping increasingly effective behavior.

Self-monitoring on a moment-by-moment, hour-by-hour, or day-by-day basis generally produces more accurate data for assessment and practice monitoring, but other more important advantages exist. Every time clients see their self-monitoring charts on the refrigerator door or bathroom mirror, they are prompted to complete the tasks they have assigned themselves. The act of monitoring some forms of undesirable actions (such as smoking) also may interrupt overlearned behavior chains and thereby allow the client additional time to consider alternative choices. A client working on choices and consequences often finds it useful to sit down at the time a choice comes up, writing down the available choices and the short- and long-term positive and negative consequences associated with each. (Writing an e-mail message to the social worker or friend spelling these out also can be helpful.) Notice that by doing one of these things, the client is practicing this new approach to life in his or her own environment.

Although practicing new social skills with the clinician is often important as a learning tool, practice in the natural environment is a crucial next step. For example, Sloane (1976/1988) has developed a procedure in which parents of teenagers practice being good listeners who encourage (rather than punish) their children to talk openly and honestly. In this process, the teenagers make up situations that the parent might not like or might be concerned about, and the parent learns to listen without interrupting, to reward honesty, to ask thoughtful questions, and to express constructive concerns. After practicing these skills in the home with one's children, it is more likely that they will then be used in real situations during similar stimulus conditions. In another example, a successful aggression-reduction program in a school involved practicing alternative behaviors around the school and self-monitoring by young people to determine how well they used new repertoires (Ninness, Ellis, Miller, Baker, & Rutherford, 1995).

The form and timing of home tasks are important. For clients who have well-established writing and record-keeping repertoires, the task of keeping charts or journals can more easily be developed. Other clients may need extensive assistance, including forms provided by the worker or follow-up telephone calls. It may be necessary to keep assignments simple in the beginning, and to develop self-management programs to support completion. Completing assignments is important for clients. It is essential that the worker ask about assignments at the beginning of the next session, provide reinforcement for completion or progress, and nonpunitively discuss effective ways to structure tasks or deal with obstacles that have come up if tasks have not been substantially completed.

Any of the interventive strategies described in earlier chapters lend themselves to the development of home tasks, including trying (or writing down options regarding) life experiments, keeping track of the use and effectiveness of efforts to change or accept private events, and identifying appropriate situations for using (and later practicing) skills rehearsed in sessions. Data collected on any of these assignments are among the most critical for monitoring the effectiveness of the interventive strategies being used. The task planning and implementation sequence discussed in chapter 3 is applicable across this entire range of tasks, because all require careful preparation if they are to be successful.

Procedural Variations

The behavioral literature suggests several variations that can be worked into skills training and that may make transfer to the natural environment more likely (Stokes & Baer, 1977; Stokes and Baer also suggest other strategies not discussed here that may be applicable to clinical situations). The most common method, labeled *train and hope* by Stokes and Baer, is to teach the client new skills and hope that those skills generalize to other settings. This is a weak approach and leaves too much to chance. A different approach that works but that can be labor-intensive is to implement the teaching procedure in each setting in which the skills would be useful. It may be more realistic, however, to give the client an opportunity to practice new skills in a range of situations, for example, with different people or under different conditions; given sufficient exemplars the new skill also may transfer to others.

A different approach is to ensure that some elements of the training situation are also present in the natural environment. For example, if effective communication behavior is taught in an office working from a wall chart listing desirable statement forms (for example, "I would prefer . . .," "I felt _____ when . . .," and "Thank you for . . ."), a client might post a similar chart at home or in the office for use at appropriate times, carry a small card with the same sentence lead-ins on it, or place such a card by the telephone. Another example would be a client who practices providing verbal reinforcers to others in role-playing situations in the office, keeping track on a golf counter that is also used in the natural environment.

MAINTAINING CHANGE

The first challenge in most clinical work (with the exception of practice focused on maintaining a particular level of functioning) is to achieve change, whether in private events such as self-talk and emotions or in other areas such as relationship skills. Just because a client has learned a new behavior, however, does not mean that the behavior will continue. Maintenance of change has proved to be a serious challenge for all practice models; behaviorists have paid considerable attention to this area in recent years. Three related but somewhat distinct approaches exist for supporting new repertoires in the client's natural world: (1) gradually fading artificial reinforcers, (2) shifting over time from artificial to natural reinforcers, and (3) designing new networks of reinforcement in the client's social environment.

Fading Artificial Reinforcement

Intermittent schedules of reinforcement (see chapter 1) tend to result in behavior that is more resistant to extinction than do continuous schedules. One common strategy for maintaining change in many types of behavioral work is to gradually fade the frequency with which reinforcement follows a behavior. There are two important considerations in doing so, however. First, there is a limit to how infrequently a schedule of reinforcers will maintain a behavior. Reinforcement cannot be faded to nothing or the behavior will eventually fade as well. The perpetual behavior intervention does not exist.

Second, fading reinforcements has limited usefulness in clinical work with adults. Although it may be useful to pay significant attention to every instance of a client's new, effective behavior in the clinical situation and then gradually do so less frequently (this tends to happen naturally in clinical work), maintenance in the session is not the purpose of the work. This kind of fading of reinforcement in the session may be of some use for maintaining the behavior in other settings as well, but attention to contingencies in the client's natural setting will nearly always be required.

Shift from Artificial to Natural Reinforcers

This maintenance strategy is more generally applicable for clinical practice than the previous one. Often the client and social worker work together to construct new repertoires that ultimately are likely to be supported in the normal course of life. During early stages a schedule of more frequent reinforcers may be needed. For example, one assertive skill is expressing appreciation to other people. In the beginning, as a client practices this, his or her performance is likely to be awkward and uncomfortable, but the worker can reinforce successive approximations on a frequent schedule and gradually assist the client to refine this repertoire. In some cases, the client also may tell friends and family members what his or her goal is and ask them to help him or her to achieve it, so they also may reinforce more frequently and directly than would ordinarily happen. Over time, as the client becomes more skilled, the assertive behavior should produce naturally reinforcing outcomes, and the need for these artificial reinforcers will decline. (Such automatic reinforcers are sometimes called *behavior traps* because the new behavior gets "trapped" by the naturally occurring contingencies.)

Sometimes the natural levels of reinforcers are inadequate to maintain positive behaviors for many people. For example, when a couple first begin courting, they tend to provide rich and varied, relatively noncontingent reinforcers. In the normal course of a relationship, unless attention is paid to maintaining adequate mutual positive exchange, the level often fades over time (because it requires effort), and the relationship may suffer. As discussed in chapter 8, it is sometimes important to build in supports for maintaining positive reciprocity, even when such supports do not feel entirely natural.

Designing Networks of Reinforcement

A gradual shift from artificial to natural reinforcers is fine as long as an adequate level of naturally occurring reinforcers is available in the client's world, but this is not always the case. When it is not, the worker may need to assist the client to expose himself or herself to or even to construct networks and cultures of reinforcement to support the desired behaviors. For example, one of my students was working in a halfway house with a young mother just coming out of prison. The client and her mother had a long history of drug abuse. If she returned to her former life after leaving the halfway house, despite excellent progress on staying drug-free and in becoming a good parent, she would be at high risk for relapse and for losing custody, which she had lost with several older children. Clearly, this client would have a better prognosis if she could embed herself in an entirely different set of contingencies that would reinforce her newly learned repertoires.

Either of two generally applicable approaches might work in this case. The worker could assist the client in connecting with an alternative network, such as the culture of a therapeutic community that could support her new skills. (Some of these communities emphasize punishment and coercion at too high a level for many clients, whereas others recognize the need to construct and support positive behaviors through reinforcement.) Alternatively, the worker and client might work together to construct a new culture in the client's natural environment, working to change patterns of mutual exchange in the client's family, connecting the client more intimately with existing positive people in her neighborhood, and working with her employer to facilitate success in employment. It is important to ensure that the natural network really does support the new repertoires. The client—or in some cases the worker—may need to ask people directly to provide such support and even to keep track for a period of when they do. A combination of exposure to new sources of social reinforcement for positive action and making changes in patterns of exchange within the client's existing networks is often a powerful strategy and is discussed in detail in chapter 9 in the section on addictions.

Up to this point, the material in this book has outlined general strategies applicable to clinical work, with most presenting issues and intervention goals. In nearly every social work case, completing an adequate individualized assessment is necessary, and this assessment should lead to collaborative selection of some subset of interventive techniques. The plan will often include some mixture of exposure to new experiences, work with private events, and skills training. In most cases the social worker needs to pay explicit attention to the transfer, and always to the maintenance, of new repertoires in the client's natural environment. The chapters that follow trace this process with regard to several clinical issues for which clients commonly consult with social workers. As is true in practice, each chapter demonstrates that to be maximally effective the social worker needs both familiarity with general theoretical principles and specific knowledge about the focal issue.

REFERENCES

Ginsburg, E. H. (1990). *Effective interventions: Applying learning theory to school social work.* New York: Greenwood Press.

Malott, R. W., Whaley, D. L., & Malott, M. E. (1993). *Elementary principles of behavior* (2nd ed.). Englewood Cliffs, NJ: Prentice Hall.

Ninness, H.A.C., Ellis, J., Miller, W. B., Baker, D., & Rutherford, R. (1995). The effect of a self-management training package on the transfer of aggression control procedures in the absence of supervision. *Behavior Modification, 19,* 464–490.

Reid, W. J. (1992). *Task strategies.* New York: Columbia University Press.

Sloane, H. N. (1988). *The good kid book.* Champaign, IL: Research Press. (Original work published 1976)

Stokes, T. F., & Baer, D. M. (1977). An implicit technology of generalization. *Journal of Applied Behavior Analysis, 10,* 349–367.

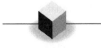

CHAPTER SEVEN

DEPRESSION AND DEMORALIZATION

M any clients consult social workers because they feel demoralized or depressed and are experiencing little or no joy. In many clinical settings, this is the most common issue social workers face. The overriding goal in these cases is to change the emotion, but emotions cannot be changed directly. The strategies for addressing this class of issues involve changes in exposure to environmental events and conditions, changes in the client's sensitivity to such conditions, and changing self-talk. The first type of change relies on a range of interventions targeting antecedents and consequences of behavior. Affecting sensitivity may include both biologically based medical treatment and behavioral work with motivating antecedents. Interventions focused on self-talk, including cognitive therapy, ultimately also result in changing exposure and sensitivity to contingencies, but indirectly.

ASSESSING DEPRESSION AND DEMORALIZATION

Depression and demoralization are not unidimensional clinical phenomena. Their complexity is perhaps reflected in the multiple *Diagnostic and Statistical Manual of Mental Disorders* (DSM)diagnoses that may be given to a client who reports being depressed, including Major Depressive Disorder, Dysthymic Disorder, bipolar disorders, "double depression" (Major Depressive Disorder superimposed on Dysthymic Disorder), Adjustment Disorder with Depressed Mood, and a number of other diagnostic codes; some of these diagnoses also include multiple additional specifiers across a range of dimensions, including chronicity and catatonic, melancholic, and seasonal features. The evidence that each of these represents a unique and separate mental illness is scant, however, and from an ecobehavioral perspective, they may perhaps be viewed best as rough descriptions of clusters of issues, rather than as discrete diagnostic entities. Whatever the diagnosis, it is still crucial to assess each client's circumstances and develop an individualized plan. A psychiatric diagnosis such as those listed above can provide a useful professional short-hand but typically provides only limited guidance for intervention. The material in this chapter is meant to be applicable across the range of clients who present as demoralized or depressed; variations depending on severity and symptom constellations are noted.

A number of tools can be useful for completing a comprehensive assessment of these issues. Any of several rapid assessment instruments can be used to do a rough screening for the presence or absence of significant depressive symptoms. The Beck Depression Inventory (Beck, Rush, Shaw, & Emery, 1978) is commonly used, for example. The items included in the Beck Depression Inventory focus on cognitive self-talk, so the instrument may be particularly helpful with clients for whom this appears to be an issue. The Generalized Contentment Scale (Hudson, 1992) is another popular instrument for screening. Standardized instruments such as these provide little specific guidance for work with an individual client (although specific item responses can suggest threads to pursue in the clinical interview) but can be useful for both quick screening and monitoring progress over time.

Behavior, especially verbal behavior, is usually the heart of assessment for depression. Motor behavior, including slowness, sad facial expressions, long latencies in responding, and slumping posture, often is the clinician's first indication of possible depression. (Substantial motor agitation also may be present, which may occasionally look like a symptom of a psychotic disorder; careful assessment of history and other symptoms may be required in such cases.) In most cases, the most important specific data will be collected in the clinical interview. The interview should include questions to assess the presence and severity of the kinds of issues listed in Figure 7-1; such questions can be comfortably interwoven within the interview.

Assessment of Suicidality

Although not all depressed or demoralized people are suicidal, most suicidal people are depressed, so in work with this group of individuals the clinician must always keep the potential for suicide in mind. Much is known about predicting risk for suicidal behavior, although one must rely on clinical judgment, because people who do not fit any standard typology commit suicide as well. All clients who talk about suicide should be taken seriously. Even

- Mood (sad, empty, depressed, irritable)
- Level of hope present
- Level of interest or pleasure experienced
- Eating patterns, weight loss or gain
- Sleep patterns
- Psychomotor agitation or retardation
- Level of energy experienced
- Sense of personal worth (a question of equivalence relations)
- Experiences of guilt
- Ability to think and concentrate
- Thoughts of death
- Thoughts of suicide
- View of one's world (self-talk)
- View of the future (self-talk)
- Family history of mood disorders and response to psychotropic medications
- Substance use and medication history
- Types and frequencies of negative experiences in the past
- Types and frequencies of negative experiences in the present
- Types and frequencies of positive experiences in the past
- Types and frequencies of positive experiences in the present
- Situations in which one feels more or less depressed

Figure 7-1. Domains to explain in assessing presence and level of depression. Criteria listed in the *DSM-IV* (American Psychiatric Association, 1994) may be helpful in determining level of depression based on intrapersonal variables listed above; complete assessment, however, requires examination of transactional exchanges as well.

those whose suicidal behavior appears manipulative often experience some ambivalence about living or dying as a result of multiple, conflicted sets of contingencies. The safest route for the social worker, if there appears to be genuine risk, is to refer the client for evaluation by a person specializing in assessment for suicide, often through a psychiatric emergency department. Every agency or private practice setting should have an established protocol for dealing with potentially suicidal clients.

Clinical Practice with Individuals

Predictors for suicide include demographic factors, personal and family history, situational factors, and current client behavior (Maris, 1992). White males, especially older white males and young adults, are at high risk for completing suicide, although women make more attempts. American Indian and inner-city African American youths are also at substantial risk. People with histories of prior attempts commonly show patterns of escalating severity, and often ultimately do complete suicide; those with a family history of suicide or who are exposed to other models are also at elevated risk. Recent losses also are important predictors. Many situational aversives are associated with suicide, including social isolation (including living alone), family and marital problems, work problems, and serious or cumulative stress. Depression, some mental illnesses, alcohol and drug abuse, and physical illness increase risk substantially.

With current behavior, hopelessness is a stronger predictor of suicide than depression. Talk about suicide or death, "termination behavior" (saying goodbye, giving away possessions), arranging to have a lethal method (drugs, a gun) available, and anger and irritability are all common in suicidal people. Certainly any client showing one or a pattern of these predictors should be regarded as at risk until suicide has been clearly ruled out. Human beings appear to be the only species that commits suicide intentionally, probably because suicide involves complex verbal processes. Later in this section, I return to this point, because it has significant implications for intervention.

If any reason exists to be concerned about the potential for suicide and if the client is communicative, the social worker should always ask whether the client has ever thought about hurting himself or herself. Asking will not "put the idea in the client's mind"; clients who are not considering suicide will say so and will appreciate the concern shown by asking. Most clinicians know this, but some find that they do not ask when they know they should. It is stressful for the worker if the client says "yes"; consequently, social workers commonly avoid asking the question. Role-played rehearsals and knowing the protocol for dealing with potential suicide situations are helpful ways to ensure that the question is asked when it needs to be.

Asking about suicide can be done naturally. In a first client contact, the worker will usually ask about depression and hopelessness as well as about major situational stressors; if there is any indication either verbally or in the client's tone of voice that suicide could be an issue, simply asking, "Have you ever thought about suicide?" or "Have you ever thought about hurting yourself?" opens the discussion in a natural way. I have never had a client act surprised or disturbed about being asked these questions, even in an initial telephone contact, and clients often express relief that it is all right to talk about such issues. Ongoing assessment of suicide potential also is important. People who have decided to kill themselves sometimes experience a real sense of relief and therefore look less depressed. Clients who are extremely depressed often lack the energy to plan a suicide, but when the depression lifts, they sometimes can do so. Suicide can be a risk if a client experiences substantial setbacks in the course of ongoing clinical work. Building a network of supports, including the social worker, family and friends, and available emergency response services is important both at the moment of acute risk and over the long-term, because working one's way out of a suicidal condition is a difficult and uneven process.

Factors Leading to and Maintaining Depression

Physiological factors may be associated with depression. It is plausible, but not certain, that some people may be prone to depression as a result of differences in the way neurotransmitters such as serotonin are produced and processed in the body. It also seems clear that life experiences can produce depression; when this happens, it does so through some kind of physiological process. At this time, no clear way is known to distinguish depressive problems for which the origin may be biological but that produce social withdrawal, irritability, and so forth from those for which the origin is in environmental events but that produce physiological sequelae.

However, many people who present as hopeless, demoralized, sad, or depressed experience few high-quality reinforcers and many serious aversives. For many of these clients, changes in the reinforcer–aversive balance is important to resolving depression. (One of the effects of medication, for example, is to increase sensitivity to available reinforcers.) For this reason, a behavioral ecomap can be an important aid to help the client and clinician identify both specific sources of reinforcement and aversives in the client's life-space, as well as overall patterns such as a lack of strong positives from anywhere in the client's social world. Figure 7-2 is an example of such a map, depicting few social reinforcers in the life of an isolated, demoralized young man.

Much is known about how environmental events may be associated with depression. (This discussion loosely follows Dougher & Hackbert, 1994). Depressed people often are inactive and therefore experience a low density of

Clinical Practice with Individuals

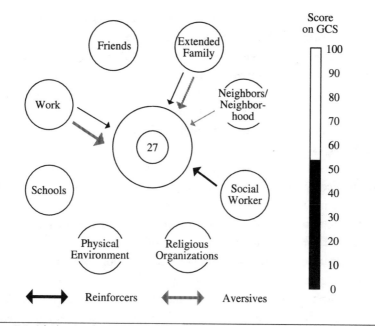

Figure 7-2. A behavioral ecomap depicting the life situation of an isolated young man who was depressed and his score on the Generalized Contentment Scale (Hudson, 1992).

high-quality reinforcers. Sometimes this situation reflects a lack of reinforcement, sometimes lack of access skills, and sometimes limitations in the social repertoires needed to make connections.

Losses of important sources of reinforcement (for example, divorce or death of a parent) can lead to extinction-related depression, particularly for people who are unable to connect with alternative sources in a reasonable time. Resolution of grief and loss requires more than finding alternative sources of reinforcers, although these are important. Resolution also often requires that the person come into contact with cues previously associated with the person (or other source of positives) who has been lost and come to accept the anger, sadness, grief, and other feelings (an exposure process). As with other negative emotions, efforts to block the experience of these emotions only prolong the pain. People's tolerance for such experience varies and as a result so does the length of time required for resolution. In the case of an intimate relationship, some pain may be experienced for a long time.

Generally unresponsive environments (as experienced by many neglected children) also can produce depressive behavior as a result of limited available reinforcement for any behavior. Prolonged and inescapable punishment (as occurs in cases of child abuse or battering) appears to lead to depression. Situations associated with aversive events in the past also are commonly avoided, and disavoidance may further reduce access to reinforcement. The physiological experience of feeling depressed can be associated with settings in which one has been depressed before; many people find that their level of depression varies between work and home because of their differential histories in each setting.

Distressed behavior associated with depression also can be shaped and maintained by the social environment (Biglan, 1991). Acting sad, crying, complaining, and other behaviors often associated with depression tend, in the short run, to be protective, because other individuals are less likely to act aggressively toward people acting that way. Others do, however, tend to act aggressively later when the person is not acting so depressed, so it is easy to see how acting in a depressed way may be in part maintained by negative reinforcement. In addition, other people tend to avoid contact with people who act depressed, consequently, their opportunities for social reinforcement are further reduced. These patterns constitute a clinical challenge, because the worker needs to communicate empathy for the pain the client is experiencing but does not want to reinforce the client primarily for depressed talk. This is a complicated issue, but in general, in the beginning an effective worker will provide a high level of empathy and reinforce the client for talking about all kinds of experiences, including those of sadness and those that are more positive. Over time, the worker will increasingly attend to healthy steps the client is taking. This change in attention is not done secretly or manipulatively. Rather, the clinician says something such as, "I really do hear how difficult this is for you. I am particularly impressed that despite those painful feelings, you have been reaching out to people in the past week. As we have talked about, taking those active steps is what will eventually make you feel better."

Cognitive therapists have observed patterns that characterize the self-talk of depressed clients. Two major types of depressive self-talk are of strong clinical relevance and tend to be interrelated. First, many depressed clients experience hopelessness that is rooted in rules that say, "There is nothing that I can do that will improve my life. Nothing can make me happy. Things will be like this forever." Given such rules, of course, it is not surprising that the client takes few active steps to change his or her situation. During such circumstances, clients often notice only those negative events and conditions that are consistent with

Clinical Practice with Individuals

their self-talk. Many clients have learned rules such as, "I want to change my life, but I am too depressed to do it. . . . It would take too much effort, and I don't have enough energy,"—clearly a self-defeating stance but one many clients have accepted as an accurate statement of the contingencies.

A second class of self-talk associated with hopelessness and depression involves equivalence relations. A client who has learned relations such as

$$\text{myself} \approx \text{depressed} \approx \text{hopeless} \approx \text{unattractive} \approx \text{failure}$$

and

$$\text{other people} \approx \text{selfish} \approx \text{uncaring}$$

and perhaps

$$\text{other people} \approx \text{smarter than me} \approx \text{happier than me}$$

is less likely to take the steps required to act in his or her world than someone who has not. Hayes (1992) has suggested that one way to understand suicide is to see that it often involves verbal associations following construction of an equivalence relation, such as

$$\text{relief} \approx \text{death} \approx \text{jumping from a bridge.}$$

The positive functions of relief therefore come to be associated with suicidal behavior.

This discussion offers a way of understanding the cognitive triad identified by cognitive therapists as usually present in depression: a negative view of oneself, a negative view of one's world (including the social world), and a negative view of the future (Beck, Rush, Shaw, & Emery, 1978). The first two views clearly involve equivalence relations, whereas the hopelessness involved in the third view is rooted in rules. Interventive strategies for addressing problems in self-talk as well as in exposure to environmental contingencies are outlined below. Notice that there are usually substantial connections among these levels. A client who experiences few positives also often believes that there is nothing he or she can do to achieve more satisfying experiences. Similarly, a client who believes himself or herself to be unpleasant or irritating to be around is unlikely to expose himself or herself to people and therefore to a potential increase in social reinforcement. Concurrent attention to both self-talk and active behavioral change is therefore often required. This requirement has been recognized both by those clinicians whose primary orientation is cognitive and by those whose primary orientation is behavioral (recall that in the ecobehavioral approach, cognitive events are viewed as a subset of behavior; see, for example, Beck, Rush, Shaw, & Emery, 1978; Ellis & Dryden, 1987). Clients are unlikely to maintain improvements in mood unless they experience genuine changes in their transactions with the physical and social environment, but it is usually necessary to address self-talk to prompt taking the active steps required to reshape one's life.

INTERVENTIVE STRATEGIES

The core process for resolving issues of depression and demoralization is to assist the client to obtain valued reinforcers and to limit contact with serious aversives. A person who is empowered to do so will typically experience only passing experiences of demoralization and substantial joy, fulfillment, and satisfaction. Obviously, this is a more difficult goal to achieve for members of oppressed and disempowered groups. Clients from such groups will often do best if they are able to connect to social networks and cultural entities in which they can begin to experience shared power (Lowery and Mattaini, 1996). Encouraging exposure to new sets of contingencies from such social networks is one of three basic interventive strategies that will be outlined below. A second approach that has substantial empirical support is work to change self-talk (cognitive therapy), which can facilitate exposure and sensitivity to new experiences. The third is referral for antidepressant medication. Each of these strategies operates at a different level (the environmental, private events, and physiological). Because of the clear connections among them, however, intervention at any one can affect the others, and a comprehensive plan involves all three. These strategies will be discussed in reverse order, building from the simple to the complex. Throughout the discussion, however, it is important to keep the goal of personal empowerment (assisting the client to act to obtain valued reinforcers and to limit contact with serious aversives) in mind.

Antidepressant Medication

Although this statement may appear odd, antidepressant medication can be a valuable tool for achieving empowerment. Antidepressant medications can, for many depressed people, increase sensitivity to environmental reinforcers and energy for taking active steps. Taking such medications can facilitate action to change one's experiences, obtain access to positive reinforcers, and minimize aversives. Some clients can benefit from a short course of antidepressant medication, experiment with new behavior that produces new outcomes (often with help from a clinician), and then discontinue the medication as their behavior comes under control of the new contingencies. Others may, for reasons probably related to the idiosyncratic ways their bodies process neurotransmitters, require medication for long periods but be better able to respond to important reinforcers when taking it. For this latter group, antidepressant medications may function in a manner analogous to insulin for people with diabetes.

Some social workers have discouraged clients from the use of antidepressant medications because of a misunderstanding of the functions of these medications or out of professional insecurity (because psychotropic medications must be prescribed by a physician). People who are severely depressed usually require medications for an adequate outcome, and discouraging a client from using medication would be an ethically questionable action. Depressed clients who show many melancholic symptoms are particularly likely to need and to benefit from antidepressant medications. Such symptoms (sometimes called "vegetative signs") include loss of pleasure in most activities or in reaction to usually pleasurable events, experiencing depression as qualitatively different from other experiences such as reactions to death, early morning awakening, depression worst in the morning, motor retardation or agitation, weight loss or anorexia, and excessive guilt (American Psychiatric Association, 1994). For other depressed clients, if nonchemical approaches do not begin to produce relief within a reasonable period (perhaps four to six weeks), consideration should be given to referral for possible medication.

Social workers should become familiar with the common classes of antidepressant medications (selective serotonin reuptake inhibitors such as fluoxetine [Prozac] and sertaline hydrochloride [Zoloft], heterocyclics such as nortriptyline [Pamelor] and amitriptyline [Elavil], and monoamine oxidase inhibitors such as phenelzine [Nardil] and tranylcypromine [Parnate]). With most antidepressant medications, clinical response is unlikely for at least two, and often several, weeks after an adequate dose is prescribed. It is common to begin with a low dose and then gradually increase the dosage. This procedure may further extend the time for a clinical response. Although most clients with serious depression will respond to one or another antidepressant medication, there is no way to know for certain which medication will work best, so it may be necessary to experiment sequentially with more than one. Clients may require substantial support during this period and need to clearly understand that lack of immediate response does not mean that their situations are hopeless.

Professionals often agree that most clients who take antidepressant medications benefit from, and often require, clinical consultation, because medication can make new behavior possible but provides no direction for actions to take or guidance and support for learning required repertoires. This consultation will frequently focus on one or both of the other strategies discussed below.

Changing Self-Talk

A second approach with solid empirical support for work with depression is cognitive therapy, which focuses on changing self-talk (often called "self-statements," "automatic thoughts," or "irrational beliefs," depending on the theorist). The central concept is that, by changing what one says to oneself, one can change how one feels. External events (A) within this paradigm evoke self-talk (B), which in turn evokes feelings (C). As Albert Ellis (1977) frequently repeats, the stoic philosopher Epictetus noted, "What disturbs people's minds is not events but their judgments on events" (p. xv). If one believes that one's circumstances are awful and hopeless, it is not surprising that one might feel demoralized. Work with self-talk focuses on examining how one describes reality, identifying disturbing distortions, and changing them.

This approach, if used by itself (which none of the major theorists do), would be too limited. If a client experiences severe aversives over and over, it is important to help him or her minimize exposure and not only work on changing how he or she thinks about it. As an extreme example, it would certainly not be ethically justifiable to help a battered woman work toward cognitively accepting her beatings instead of at least considering other options. In addition, biological research suggests that the ABC paradigm is not an accurate description of some instances of emotional upset; in some cases nerve impulses stimulated by external events are routed directly to primitive, emotional parts of the brain without traveling to the cerebral cortex where verbal and cognitive processes occur. For people with significant biochemical imbalances (shortages of serotonin, for example), the root of the problem is not necessarily cognitive. However, even with these limitations, changing self-talk can be a powerful intervention, sometimes alone and sometimes in conjunction with other techniques (as dictated by individualized assessment).

Clinical Practice with Individuals

Although many varieties of cognitive treatment are used, they have much in common. In the sections that follow, I will outline three approaches. The first two specify in clear behavioral terms strategies used in standard cognitive therapy. The third set of techniques, from acceptance and commitment therapy (Hayes & Wilson, 1994), represents a major new direction in behavioral and cognitive–behavioral work (Hayes, Jacobson, Follette, & Dougher, 1994).

Shaping Accurate Observations, Descriptions, and Rules. Depressive self-talk often involves distortions in the way reality is observed and described, including inaccurate descriptions of the contingencies present (rules). Inaccurate observations often involve selective attention to negative events (or to negative details—*selective abstraction*) or misinterpretation of neutral or even positive events as negative. (Many of the terms used here were first used by Beck, Rush, Shaw, & Emery, 1978 and Ellis & Dryden, 1987.) These patterns can become habitual once clients begin to describe them to themselves. Distorted descriptions of reality include overgeneralizing, magnifying (for example "awfulizing"), minimizing, or overpersonalizing events. Inaccurate rules sometimes involve personal disempowerment such as "This is how it is, and there's nothing I can do about it" or "I can't stand this." In other cases they involve misperceptions or exaggerations of likely consequences of behavior, for example, "If I ask someone to have coffee with me, he or she will just laugh at me" or "I must do everything perfectly or no one will respect me."

The goal in all of these cases is to help the client observe and describe reality in accurate terms. Although some research suggests that people who have a positively distorted view of reality may be happier than those with an accurate view, I suspect this may be a matter of interpretation. At any rate, true clinical collaboration depends on honesty. It is often especially valuable to assign the homework task of noting and writing down as many events and experiences that are positive, beautiful, or in other ways worth appreciating as possible. This assignment can prompt a profound change in observational behavior and, although simple, is among the most powerful tools in work with depression.

Several basic clinical directions can be taken to help toward a goal of accurate self-talk. The most direct, which is rooted in Beck's collaborative empiricism, is to work with the client to examine the evidence for distorted statements. In effect, one is helping clients see their beliefs and self-talk as hypotheses to be tested rather than proven facts. This can be done in the session by using a Socratic dialogue such as the following:

Client (sadly): Nothing I do ever works out right . . .

Social worker: You say "nothing." I wonder if that is true. Can you think of some times when you succeeded?

Client: No, I never really do . . .

Social worker: You told me earlier that your child is doing well in school and socially and that you raised him yourself. . . . Is there some success in there?

Client: Well, I guess . . .

Social worker: How about in other areas?

Client: Well, my boss seems to put up with me . . .

Social worker: I'm not sure, but there might be a pattern here; you seem to really notice things you do wrong, but to minimize what you do right. . . . Is that true?

In this exchange, the worker is helping the client evaluate the evidence for an overgeneralized statement and to interrupt a pattern of inaccurate description of reality. Notice that it was done here in a questioning, tentative manner. If the worker used rational disputation (emphasized by Ellis), a slightly more confrontational technique, he or she might have begun (in a more friendly, warm tone) by saying, "You say 'nothing.' Sorry, I don't buy it! Your son is doing well in school, you have a good job . . . could you be overgeneralizing here—again?" Notice that the difference is one of degree, rather than quality; in the first example the worker acts more as a co-explorer; in the second, more as an expert observer sharing his or her observations. This continuum is in part a matter of personal style and may vary from client to client and situation to situation, depending on the needs of the case (experimentation may be necessary to determine where on the continuum to work).

Another dimension of collaborative empiricism is testing self-talk to determine how accurately it captures reality. This testing can sometimes be done in the session by asking questions to further explore client statements:

Social worker: You say no one cares about you . . . thinking about your family, people you know, people you work with . . . might any of them care a little? Would anyone help you if you needed it?

Client: Well, I suppose my mother would try to—but she'd also want to take control . . .

Social worker: So she does care about you, even though her way of showing it may not be just what you would prefer. Anyone else . . . ?

Clinical Practice with Individuals

The idea here is to help the client view the nuances of his or her social world—not an unrealistically positive one but an accurate one. During such discussions, clearer views of how clients would like their lives to be will also often emerge. The worker may then move with the client to explore ways to reshape the client's reality to more closely approximate the desired state. The client's view of how the world "should" or "must" be can also be profitably explored, as in the following exchange:

Client: I can't stand living alone; I'm so miserable and lonely . . . really a pathetic figure . . . .

Social worker: You say you "can't stand" living alone. What does that mean, that you'll die of loneliness?

Client: No, I guess not; I'd just be miserable forever . . . .

Social worker: So to be happy, you *must* be living with someone?

Client: Yeah.

Social worker: Why?

Client: Well, everyone needs someone in their life.

Social worker: Some people certainly are happy when they do have someone. Of course, some are pretty miserable living with someone, too. Is it really true that everyone who lives alone is miserable?

Client(tentatively): Um . . . well, maybe not everyone . . .

Depending on how the dialogue develops from here, the worker may help the client consider the possibility that he or she may be able to live alone happily. Another alternative that could be valuable during these circumstances would be to ask the client to test his or her hypothesis in life:

Social worker: How many people do you know who live alone?

Client: Quite a few, it's a lonely world out there.

Social worker: I'd like to suggest an experiment. Do you know at least six people who have lived alone for a while, like more than a few months? Yes? OK, I'd like you to ask at least six people like that if they are always miserable living alone. That's the question, "Are you always miserable living alone?" Would you be willing to do that?

Client: I guess . . .

Depression and Demoralization   111

If the client completes this task, he or she is likely to obtain a range of responses; that is exactly the point, to help him or her to be able to say, based on the evidence, that one is not always miserable when living alone. Then the intervention would typically move toward developing tasks that could enrich the client's life (see the last section of this chapter).

Work with Equivalence Relations. Many depressed clients, as discussed above, have learned equivalence relations such as

$$me \approx worthless \approx hopeless \approx undesirable \approx fat \ and \ ugly,$$
$$people \approx selfish \approx uncaring,$$
$$the \ future \approx bleak.$$

While those relations persist, whenever the client thinks about himself or herself or looks in the mirror the words that come to mind may be "fat and ugly"; whenever someone asks about the future, he or she may think "bleak." Because such relations sometimes date from childhood, were often shaped by authoritative people such as parents, and have often been practiced many, many times, simply disputing them may be inadequate. (You may have noticed that if you say to someone, "No, you're not fat!" you may often get a response like, "Yes, I am!" The equivalence relation involved is extensively modeled and reinforced in contemporary culture, which often gives the destructive message that one must be paper thin and look 17 years old to be beautiful.)

Research on equivalence relation formation is new, and the material in this section therefore tentative. Research suggests, however, that there is no simple way to dissolve an equivalence relation once it is formed. Rather, people need to form, and be reinforced for forming, alternative relations. For example, if you tell someone "You're not fat," this may function as a punisher, so the person may no longer say that in your presence, but the relation probably persists. Instead, the person probably needs to learn to form an alternative relation, for example,

$$me \approx beautiful \ in \ my \ own \ way,$$

and needs to practice and reinforce that relation in the client's life situation. (If it is reinforced only in the social worker's office, the office may serve as an occasion evoking the new relation, but other situations may continue to evoke the old one—the behavior will have come under contextual control.) Assignments similar to those suggested above also may be useful to test new equivalence relations in vivo. It may be helpful, for example, to ask the client to practice saying "people are sometimes (warm/thoughtful/kind)" and to write down or report back evidence that this is true.

Acceptance and Commitment Therapy. Another emerging behavioral approach to work with emotional struggles is acceptance and commitment therapy (ACT) (Hayes & Wilson, 1994). (ACT can be described as a cognitive–behavioral approach. In the view of its developers and this author, however, cognitive events are a subset of behavior, and the term *cognitive–behavioral* is redundant; Thyer, 1992.) Not all aspects of ACT will be discussed here, including the use of paradox and "creative hopelessness," which may give a noncollaborative message unless the social worker is well trained in their use. The core acceptance and commitment techniques, however, are widely applicable.

People who have depression (or other undesirable emotions such as anxiety or anger) often punish themselves and try to fight the emotion ("I shouldn't feel depressed"). This reaction can result in a second-order problem that sometimes can usefully be described to clients as "being depressed about being depressed" or "anxious about being anxious." From an ecobehavioral perspective, this anxiety is an obvious problem. The visceral, verbal, and motor behaviors that constitute depression (or anxiety) are just that, behaviors. They are, therefore, shaped by their antecedents and consequences. That is, unpleasant emotions are the natural result of the client's experiences. In other words, given the client's biological makeup, learning history, and current experiences, he or she should be depressed. Controlling feelings under such circumstances is therefore an impossible task, rather like trying to talk the wind out of blowing. If clients fail to control their feelings then punish themselves, the situation is only exacerbated.

Many things are best accepted, including events from the past and unchangeable aspects of reality. An important form of acceptance in work with unpleasant emotions involves being willing (not happy, but willing) to experience feelings as they come for now and for the moment. A man whose life partner has just left him for someone else is likely to experience some mix of hurt, rejection, abandonment, anger, and loneliness; his first task is to accept these feelings as they come and be willing to feel what he does. To do that, he needs to learn to observe emotions as they occur, as an objective observer, rather than to avoid them. (Hayes & Wilson, 1994, described this process as learning to discriminate the observing self from the experiencing self.)

Desensitization and action (see below) can gradually help attenuate the emotions but only if the feelings are allowed to emerge. One of the social worker's tasks, therefore, is to give the client a message such as the following:

Of course you are sad and hurt! Those are your natural reactions to what's happened in your life, and even though having those feelings is painful, it's important to allow yourself to feel them. If you can let yourself feel, you will eventually feel better. If you try to fight your emotions, they will keep coming back. There are also active steps you can take that will—eventually—help.

The active steps mentioned are the commitment aspect of acceptance and commitment. Essentially, the client determines a direction that will ultimately result in increased personal satisfaction and commits to completing the tasks required regardless of how he or she feels. Instead of saying something such as, "I'd like to go back to school, *but* I am too depressed," the client practices saying, "I'd like to go back to school, *and* I am very depressed." By substituting "and" for "but," the emotion no longer is defined as an insurmountable obstacle but as a concomitant occurrence. In this case, the client and worker would identify the steps required if the client is to go back to school, and the client would commit to taking them, even if he or she is feeling very depressed while doing so. The client is committing here to follow a rule, and the ultimate positive outcome (which will probably include feeling better emotionally) may be delayed as the result of many small cumulative steps. The client may need extensive immediate reinforcement from the worker or others in his or her environment, as well as self-management techniques, to follow through.

The active steps will usually involve exposing oneself to new sets of contingencies and experimenting with life to discover new sources of reinforcement. Ultimate resolution of depression and demoralization will usually require immersion in a different matrix of events, in particular, reducing exposure to aversive factors and increasing exposure to reinforcers. Experimentation may be required to discover how to achieve this reinforcement best. The next section of the chapter outlines several useful strategies for such experiments. In each case, many of the general interventive strategies discussed in previous chapters, such as skills training or work with private events, may be important adjuncts for achieving success.

Exposure to New Contingencies

Feeling better requires experiencing better. The real functions of medication and work with private events are to increase sensitivity to reinforcers and decrease sensitivity to aversives and to facilitate action that will result in experiencing better outcomes and more reinforcing consequences. A person who experiences high levels of fulfillment and satisfaction will not be demoralized, particularly when the positives experienced are consequences of the person's own behavior. The ecobehavioral approach defines personal empowerment in this way; the empowered person acts to influence his or her world to achieve valued outcomes and knows he or she can do so. Effective action of this kind, as recognized in the empowerment literature (Gutierrez, 1990; Simon, 1994), often requires membership in a cultural entity, a social collective that works together to achieve shared power. Assisting the client to connect with such networks is often an important aspect of clinical work. (Power is not, despite strongly overlearned cultural beliefs, limited. Real power is collective power, the result of sharing, not competition; members of more competitive cultures have much to learn from American Indian cultures in this regard; Lowery & Mattaini, 1996.)

Reinforcer Sampling. Many people who have been demoralized and depressed for long periods have little experience with potential reinforcers, and a first task for many such clients is to experiment with exposing themselves to new or forgotten sources of fulfillment. This is one variation of *reinforcer sampling*, in which a client takes opportunities to test one or more possible sources of reinforcement with the hope that some will prove to be of value. These opportunities may include recreational or cultural activities, social activities, arts, or hobbies. Often, depressed people do not experience much satisfaction in activities in the beginning so it may be necessary to encourage them to try something that they used to like or that there is reason to think they might like more than once to give it a fair chance. This is especially true if the client feels initial discomfort in new situations. I sometimes suggest that clients go on a "reinforcer hunt"; they leave their house for a few hours and explore, talk to people, go to a movie and a bookstore, or do other activities until they find something satisfying. It is possible to accomplish this task at home, by doing several things (for example, calling a friend, listening to music, or cooking) until something is experienced as pleasant. The hunt metaphor is useful here, because although not every hunt is successful, the hunter keeps trying until something is caught.

Activity Scheduling. Activity scheduling is valuable for clients who tend not to plan ahead and therefore have few positive experiences. In early stages, the social worker helps the client identify a few things that he or she might find satisfying and could do in the next few days. The client is then asked to schedule these activities and to treat them as important appointments that should be kept. Making such a commitment is important for clients who have difficulty in getting started or who may tell themselves that they do not deserve to engage in positive activities out of guilt or as a result of irrational self-talk.

Choosing activities is sometimes simple, but often it is not. When clients cannot identify any promising alternatives, the clinician may provide the rationale that in the beginning, practicing taking any kind of action is the most important consideration and it does not matter so much what is done or whether it is immediately satisfying. As noted above, it may take several exposures before the positive effects of an activity are experienced, so commitment techniques can be crucial to break through to more positive experiences.

Choices and Consequences. The procedures in choices and consequences were outlined in chapter 4. In work with depressed clients, this strategy can be particularly empowering because it can help overcome hopelessness and demoralization. Given the client's current situation, available choices for increasing access to reinforcers and decreasing exposure to aversive factors can be outlined, then followed by thoughtful analysis of the probable long- and short-term consequences of each. A behavioral ecomap may be helpful in this process to capture the client's overall contextual situation and to identify potential action points.

Social contacts, positive and aversive, are among the most powerful events for shaping human behavior, including emotions, probably because of the evolutionary advantages to people who were members of supportive social groups such as families and clans. In most cases of depression, demoralization, or alienation, a scan of patterns of social impacts on the client identifies few high-quality social reinforcers, a high level of social aversives, or both. These interpersonal deficits and excesses are often crucial foci for intervention. In fact, another form of treatment for depression with strong empirical

Clinical Practice with Individuals

support is *interpersonal psychotherapy* (Klerman & Weissman, 1982), which emphasizes resolution of relationship difficulties, including role disputes (which often involve substantial aversive exchange), role transitions (which involve learning to acquire adequate reinforcers under new conditions), interpersonal deficits (skills deficits and, in some cases, problems of faulty discriminations), and grief (which involves extinction). Although interpersonal psychotherapy emerged largely from psychodynamic theory, it is easy to understand, in behavioral terms, why it should be effective in many cases.

Many of the other interpersonal strategies found elsewhere in this book (especially in the next chapter) can be useful to help clients take the steps needed to change their social experiences. Choices and consequences, often in combination with other interventive strategies as described above, is a particularly useful strategy for addressing such issues, to develop alternative plans to access better-quality or more frequent social positives, or to think through ways to limit exposure to aversives. For example, an isolated, lonely, demoralized young man seen by the author considered the options of taking classes, joining a wrestling club and a literary discussion group (in each of which social interaction is structured into the activity in a routine way), and exploring job opportunities that would offer more human contact than his current work cataloguing manuscripts in a library. Each option had costs of various kinds associated with it, and some involved more social risks than others. Recognizing that he had options, however, was an important first step.

Another client, a depressed young woman, also was socially isolated and also was in regular phone and sometimes face-to-face contact with "a torturing ex"—a long-time boyfriend who was consistently emotionally abusive toward her. Although they had broken up several weeks before, it was clear that for each of them the other was still a central figure. The client reported that her few friends and family kept telling her she should not speak with him again and she had often "decided" not to. However, when she became very lonely, she would contact him, or take his calls, and not tell others she was doing so. Choices and consequences was helpful to her in several ways; first, to establish that there were several options available in terms of level, type, and frequency of contacts and how to deal with those that went wrong and, second, to help her understand what she was getting from the relationship and the consequences that were maintaining her current behavior.

She wondered whether she was somehow seeking the pain involved, but with very little work it became clear how tremendously aversive being alone was to her and that the intimacy and contact she did get from her ex-boyfriend helped relieve this. Her behavior, in other words, was functional; it was also emotionally costly. Currently, she is experimenting with trying to build other, alternative emotional connections at the same time she is trying to manage contacts with her ex-boyfriend more thoughtfully and assertively. She recognizes that she has choices and that making a particular choice often involves a mix of positive and negative, short- and long-term consequences. This strategy can be powerful. Use of graphic tools such as the choices and consequences matrix shown in Figure 4-1 (p. 59) can often facilitate the process.

Environmental Intervention. It is advantageous to encourage and support clients to take the necessary steps to expose themselves to new environmental contingencies. Experiencing the positive effects of one's own actions is empowering. Certain clients, however, lack the essential repertoires required to make some changes. Many clients with severe mental illness, for example, can take some steps on their own but also may need direct assistance from the social worker to locate and access better living conditions. Some depressed people do not have the skills or energy required to resolve some interpersonal conflicts without direct intervention by the clinician. Many depressed clients are in long-conflicted family or work relationships in which coercive exchange and aversive stimulation are firmly established. In such cases, part of the responsibility of the social worker is to actively engage the client's environment by working conjointly with clients and other family members or by mediating a conflict at the client's place of employment as examples.

Where events and conditions in the social and physical environment are major roots of the depression or demoralization experienced by a client, the first preference is to help the client act to make changes, using some combination of these techniques. Where the client lacks either the basic repertoires required or access to important actors, the clinician often must take direct action to help arrange a situation in which the client is in a position to act to obtain a higher level of reinforcement or a lower level of aversives. All of this can be extremely challenging, especially because many of the clients seen in clinical practice are seriously demoralized. Such clients certainly need rapid success in some area, and the social worker may need, in the early stages, to help arrange for adequate reinforcement for clients' efforts, even when they may not yet be as consistent or skillful as they may become later. Thinking through alternative environmental access points in a truly ecobehavioral way is an important first step, followed by collaborative work with the client to determine who should do what to make substantive changes in the overall configuration.

REFERENCES

American Psychiatric Association. (1994). *Diagnostic and statistical manual of mental disorders* (4th ed.). Washington, DC: American Psychiatric Association.

Beck, A. T., Rush, A. J., Shaw, B. F., & Emery, G. (1978). *Cognitive therapy of depression.* New York: Guilford Press.

Biglan, A. (1991). Distressed behavior and its context. *Behavior Analyst, 14,* 157–169.

Dougher, M. J., & Hackbert, L. (1994). A behavior-analytic account of depression and a case report using acceptance-based procedures. *Behavior Analyst, 17,* 321–334.

Ellis, A. (1977). *Anger: How to live with and without it.* Secaucus, NJ: Citadel.

Ellis, A., & Dryden, W. (1987). *The practice of rational-emotive therapy.* New York: Springer.

Gutierrez, L. M. (1990). Working with women of color: An empowerment perspective. *Social Work, 35,* 149–153.

Hayes, S. C. (1992). Verbal relations, time and suicide. In S. C. Hayes & L. J. Hayes (Eds.), *Understanding verbal relations* (pp. 109–118). Reno, NV: Context Press.

Hayes, S. C., Jacobson, N. S., Follette, V. M., & Dougher, M. J. (Eds.). (1994). *Acceptance and change: Content and context in psychotherapy.* Reno, NV: Context Press.

Hayes, S. C., & Wilson, K. G. (1994). Acceptance and commitment therapy: Altering the verbal support for experiential avoidance. *Behavior Analyst, 17,* 289–303.

Hudson, W. W. (1992). *WALMYR assessment scales scoring manual.* Tempe, AZ: WALMYR.

Klerman, G. L., & Weissman, M. M. (1982). Interpersonal psychotherapy: Theory and research. In A. J. Rush (Ed.), *Short-term psychotherapies for depression* (pp. 88–106). New York: Guilford Press.

Lowery, C. T., & Mattaini, M. A. (1996). *The use of power in social work.* Unpublished manuscript.

Maris, R. W. (1992). Overview of the study of suicide assessment and prediction. In R. W. Maris, A. L. Berman, J. T. Maltsberger, & R. I. Yufit (Eds.), *Assessment and prediction of suicide* (pp. 3–22). New York: Guilford Press.

Simon, B. L. (1994). *The empowerment tradition in American social work: A history.* New York: Columbia University Press.

Thyer, B. A. (1992). The term "cognitive–behavior therapy" is redundant. *Behavior Therapist, 15*(5), 112, 128.

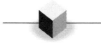

CHAPTER EIGHT

RELATIONSHIP ISSUES

Positive social exchanges may be the strongest elements shaping and enriching human life; aversive and coercive social exchanges are among the deepest sources of human pain. Because human beings are by nature social, relationship disruptions and social deprivation can have profound effects on their lives. Social workers' efforts to enhance relationships occur at many system levels, from family and group work to community practice to policy analysis and advocacy. Although it is often an advantage to work concurrently with the many people involved in relationship issues or to work in a group that offers multiple and varied opportunities to practice new repertoires, relationship difficulties affect many clients seen individually. Deficits and excesses in social behavior often result in severe isolation (and loneliness), and many clients seen individually identify improvements in relationships among their most important goals.

CULTURE AND RELATIONSHIPS

Cultural differences are particularly relevant in relationship issues. In this book, "culture" refers to interlocking practices and systems of reinforcers that are maintained by a social group. This is a broad definition, encompassing phenomena from family cultures to ethnic cultures. Effective social repertoires must be defined within the interlocking cultures in which the client lives—not a simple matter. For example, certain Latino and Asian American cultures regard assertive behavior, as commonly defined in European American cultures, as inappropriate for a young woman toward her father. Some families and ethnic cultures value "connectedness" more than others that emphasize individuation. The client and worker may often need to carefully and collaboratively assess what repertoires (behaviors) the client needs to use to achieve positive results (consequences) under what circumstances (antecedents). Participating in this process requires that the worker be aware of the cultures (family, professional, religious, and ethnic) that have shaped his or her own behaviors (including beliefs) and the extent to which these may be inconsistent with those experienced by the client.

Given the importance of these cultural issues, sensitive decisions must be made in clinical planning. For example, even if assertive behavior is not consistent with the existing culture of a family, the client may still need to learn assertive skills. The worker and client may and often do determine that introducing a potentially unsettling change into the family is important to the client and may produce better outcomes for all concerned. If this decision is made, the worker should determine whether a potential for emotional or physical danger exists for the client. The worker also should recognize that for some time, people outside the family (the worker, friends, or members of support groups) may need to provide reinforcers for the new behaviors.

Bicultural or multicultural people often use different repertoires under differing antecedent conditions. For example, an American Indian who spends time on the reservation as well as in an urban setting is exposed to two dramatically different settings. The individual may need to learn different repertoires for each, and the social worker and client may need to work with members of each culture to determine the skills required and to shape the often subtle dimensions. At the same time, some repertoires should remain consistent, including the covert self-definitions that constitute "identity." Other behaviors may be reinforced in one setting but punished in another. In minor areas, this may not be aversive, but in more significant areas it can be. In the example of the American Indian, within many Indian cultures direct, honest communication is highly valued. An American Indian operating within an organizational or academic culture that rewards indirect and often manipulative communication may find the dissonance highly aversive. Under such circumstances, these individuals often find that they achieve the greatest satisfaction and the best outcomes by acting in ways consistent with who they are—repertoires shaped by their primary cultures (Lowery, in press).

Immigrants also face complicated decisions about to what extent and under what circumstances to act in ways consistent with contemporary North American culture and to what extent to maintain traditional cultural practices. For such clients, learning new skills should be presented and viewed as giving them more options rather than reshaping who they must be. A recent immigrant from Japan may decide to act assertively under some circumstances of social conflict but decide in other situations that he or she does not wish to be assertive; the social worker should respect this decision as the client's right.

Given these complexities, the material that follows should be viewed as offering strategic options for assisting clients to make changes that they desire to make in relationships. The clinician must recognize his or her own values regarding relationships and understand how these values shape what the worker sees, and values, in clients. The following are values that tend to be supported by available data, all factors being equal:

- Although there is tremendous variation among cultures at all levels, social exchanges rooted in mutual reinforcement are generally preferable to the use of aversives, even subtle ones. This value is consistent with the substantial available empirical data.
- Some of the reinforcers exchanged within close relationships should probably be provided contingently, and some, noncontingently. Doing everything for someone else without reciprocation can lead to exploitation; ultimately, relationships in which reciprocation is holistic rather than quid pro quo on a moment-to-moment basis may provide the greatest satisfaction and security.
- Honesty provides the data needed to identify probable consequences of behavior. All factors being equal (among multiple cultures they sometimes are not), I tend to encourage honesty in my work with clients. Exceptions occur (the person who had an affair 30 years ago should ordinarily not reveal this fact to a spouse when one of them is about to die, for example), but the disrespect communicated by and damage that can result from deception can lead to negative relationship outcomes.

DIMENSIONS OF RELATIONSHIP ISSUES

As shown in Figure 8-1, problems in the social and relationship areas can be envisioned as occurring within a three-dimensional space (behavior X occasion x consequence). In some cases, the main clinical challenge is to teach clients new repertoires (as in teaching assertive behaviors). With other clients, the primary focus may be on helping clients use different behaviors on appropriate occasions. With still other clients, the goal may be exposure to

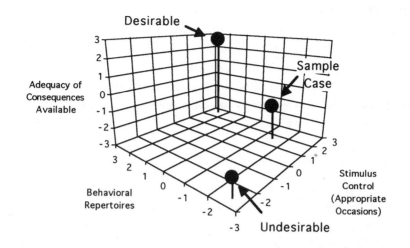

Figure 8-1. The three-dimensional space within which social behavior occurs. In the most desirable situation, the client has the required repertoires available, those behaviors occur on appropriate occasions, and they produce adequately reinforcing consequences. In the sample case shown, the client has somewhat limited repertoires (for example, assertive skills); the repertoires she has tend to occur on appropriate occasions, but the level of available social payoffs is low. This case involves deficits in behavioral repertoires and environmentally available consequences but strength in terms of appropriate stimulus control. (Sensitivity to available and socially sanctioned consequences could also be considered as a fourth dimension, which could be portrayed using different-sized spheres if desired.) Adapted with permission from Follette, W. C., Bach, P. A., & Follette, V. M. (1993). A behavior-analytic view of psychological health. *Behavior Analyst, 16*, 303–316.

more rewarding social networks (consequences). In most cases, some combination of work in this three-dimensional space may be required to achieve adequate outcomes. Relationships by definition involve the interlocking behavior of more than one person, and the behavior of one person often acts as an important antecedent or consequence of the other. Commonly, the worker and client examine these connections to develop an adequate plan, which may involve learning how to encourage others to act toward the client in different ways.

Deficits in social and relationship skills often limit the client's access to reinforcers. Approaches are available for assisting clients to use their skills on appropriate occasions (bring them under appropriate stimulus control). Many excesses of social behavior are in this category; a person may need to take aggressive action during life-threatening circumstances but the same behavior directed toward a partner or employer is a problem. Exposure to social networks that reinforce new repertoires is crucial (refer to the extensive coverage of this strategic direction in earlier chapters). Violence (among intimates and otherwise) is too complicated to be comprehensively examined here; however, a brief discussion is provided. Given its prevalence and severe negative effects on relationships, every social worker must be sensitized to the possible presence of violence and have skills for assessing and working with those individuals affected.

LEARNING RELATIONSHIP REPERTOIRES

A wide range of social repertoires can be useful for clients, including those that have sometimes been called "assertive skills," "communications skills," "social skills," and "conversation skills." Brief descriptions of a number of these follow, which may be helpful in identifying deficits for clinical focus. Decisions about which skills to emphasize must be made by the client, with attention to what is likely to produce positive outcomes and be acceptable within the client's cultural matrix. Some potentially useful skills are often underemphasized and may be extremely valuable—expressing appreciation and other forms of social reinforcement is an important example. The material in this section begins with a partial list of social repertoires that are often the focus of clinical work. The following section outlines techniques that help clients to learn these skills.

Useful Repertoires

Providing Social Reinforcers. Perhaps the most valuable social skill is providing attention, recognition, or affection to others when they act positively. Dale Carnegie recognized the importance of this principle when he wrote "give honest and sincere appreciation" (Carnegie, 1936/1981, p. 31). Finding aspects of another's behavior that can be sincerely appreciated is usually not difficult—if one looks (false praise is likely to sound patronizing and be counterproductive). Increasing the frequency of such actions is the closest thing to magic in interpersonal relationships. Many clients need both to increase the rate of social reinforcers provided and to refine how they do so to achieve maximum effect. Smiling is a universal social reinforcer, and when appropriate, touch can be powerful.

Determining when to provide reinforcers is a challenge. Early in relationships, during the "courting" stage, people tend to provide many reinforcers and limit aversives. Over time, because providing social reinforcement involves effort, it is common for the rate of positive exchange to decline, and it may be necessary to plan for maintaining it. In strong relationships, people provide reinforcers both contingent on the other person's actions (when the other does something you like and appreciate) and freely (giving a hug for no reason), with the expectation that, in the long run, such exchanges will even out. In severely conflicted relationships, each person often waits for the other to do something pleasing first—a prescription for trouble. In behavioral couples work, Stuart (1980) suggested the "change first" principle, in which each partner agrees to increase positive reinforcement independently, regardless of whether the other immediately reciprocates. This framework can be useful for increasing positive exchange in many types of relationships, because others tend to reciprocate positive as well as negative reinforcement.

The form of effective social reinforcers varies from culture to culture. Saying "thank you" and giving compliments directly are generally effective, as are more subtle actions such as finding something in what the other person says to agree with, smiling, or asking thoughtful questions. In some ethnic, geographic, or family cultures in some relationships respectful silence and attention may be more appropriate. Social workers should obtain as much knowledge and experience among cultures as possible to make it easier to determine what will work for clients in their situations. Ultimately, of course, what is reinforcing and what increases the frequency of a behavior, is an empirical question.

Accepting Social Reinforcers. Many clients and other people have not learned how to accept sincere praise and appreciation graciously. As a result, they fail to reinforce those who reinforce them. A sincere, pleased, "thank you," (perhaps followed by "I'm glad you like it" or "I'm glad you found it helpful") delivered with eye contact is a good start but can feel uncomfortable for many until practiced. Embarrassment or excessive humility can embarrass the initiator in turn, and an excessive show of pride also can put the other person off. Clients can practice with workers until they feel comfortable accepting sincere praise (see below for further detail regarding such rehearsal).

Applying Listening Skills. Knowing how to listen to other people in a respectful way is among the most critical of social skills and is often one with which clients struggle. The first step in listening, which may seem obvious but is uncommon, is to sit quietly and pay attention to what the other person is saying without interrupting or thinking about how to respond. Nonverbal signs of attention (for example, eye contact in many, but not all, cultures) are important and may need to be practiced. Furthering responses (for example, "I see" or "Um-hmm") and questions that are real requests for more information rather than veiled statements or criticisms (for example, "Did you go with that strange woman?") can reinforce the other person for talking and help maintain a positive conversational flow. Most people appreciate it when someone else listens to them; listening is often an important skill for men to learn, because in American culture, many men have not learned to listen respectfully, especially to women.

Showing Empathy. There are two aspects of empathy: feeling what the other is feeling and communicating that one does so. The second skill is easier to learn. Active listening skills, in which the listener paraphrases what the speaker says and is feeling ("It sounds like it was painful for you to hear that"), and thoughtful open-ended questions are particularly useful as are nonverbal skills such as quiet attention and appropriate body language. These skills can often be taught to clients relatively easily (see Gordon, 1970).

Helping clients to be empathic, to experience emotions similar to those experienced by another person, is more difficult because a technology for doing so has not been clearly explicated or tested. The worker therefore may need to use folk wisdom such as asking the client how he or she might feel during circumstances similar to another person's, which might be enhanced through covert rehearsal (rehearsing in the imagination; see below). Asking about situations when the client has experienced similar events also may be helpful. Substantial prompting, shaping, and reinforcement from the worker are likely to be required in this process.

Expressing Feelings (Both Positive and Negative). One definition of assertiveness is "interpersonal expressiveness in both positive and negative contexts" (Rakos, 1991, p. 15). Expressing feelings effectively is important for deepening and maintaining relationships. Expression of positive feelings (for example, "I am thrilled with how this project is working out" or " I have enjoyed this conversation") sometimes functions as a direct social reinforcer and in other cases results in the speaker being perceived as a "positive person," someone with whom others like to spend time. Expressing negative feelings (for example, "I was really disappointed when you didn't show up") rather than attributing blame to someone else ("You are so thoughtless! How could you leave me standing there by myself?") can facilitate problem resolution rather than the

Clinical Practice with Individuals

escalation of conflict. In the last example, the speaker is punishing the listener; punishment, as noted in earlier chapters, often results in counteraggression and damage to the relationship. Stating one's feelings is a way of being honest without punishing. Note that "I" statements (statements beginning with the word "I" followed by the specification of a feeling) are effective ways to express both positive and negative emotions. Many clients do not express feelings often and at first may be uncomfortable doing so. Practice is important, both in the session and as homework.

Expressing Opinions. Besides feelings, people have opinions, and effective expression of opinions is an important skill. Some clients do not express their thoughts often and as a result may be left out of conversations; others express their opinions as if they were facts, which often puts others off. Both patterns are the result of previous learning history. Practice in stating one's thoughts without experiencing excessive punishment and gradually learning to experience others' disagreements as tolerable are important for the first group of clients. For the second group, learning to begin with, "I think . . ." and to use a less demanding tone and less aggressive body language are often critical components.

Providing Appropriate Personal Disclosure. What to disclose about oneself and one's life in social situations is a complicated matter. Clients often must learn that some disclosures are appropriate with certain audiences but not with others; they must learn to recognize appropriate occasions (see below). Acknowledging one's mistakes and shortcomings is important to avoiding and resolving conflict, but many people do not do this effectively. Mutual discussions about life experiences are a valuable way to deepen social connections but require effective timing and a social rhythm that may require extensive rehearsal. An acceptable balance between discussion of positive experiences and complaints is also important. The client who lacks these repertoires may be viewed socially as a self-absorbed bore, someone to be avoided, or merely an audience who listens to others.

Entering and Maintaining Conversations. Socially isolated clients often have difficulty entering conversations and maintaining them. Entering conversations in part is an assertive repertoire, but many clients also need practice in knowing what to say. An important consideration here is selecting content; clients often find it important in the beginning to plan ahead, perhaps selecting topics from the newspaper or a magazine. Experimenting with ways to bring up subjects ("Did you see the piece in the *Times* this morning about . . .") and effective ways to comment on them is often required before these skills can be comfortably used. Another useful repertoire for many clients is asking others about their interests and opinions and demonstrating interest in those (for example, by asking follow-up questions).

Accepting Constructive Feedback. Clients with a substantial history of punishment often have difficulty in listening to feedback from others about how, for example, the client's behavior affected the other person without being defensive and without provoking the speaker. (It can be useful to learn to ask for such feedback.) As in many other areas, practice will often reduce the aversiveness of these situations; clients also may need inoculation training (see chapter 5) to listen to feedback (especially critical feedback).

Providing Constructive Feedback. Clients may struggle with two potential deficits in providing constructive feedback to others. Some clients provide no feedback at all, possibly leaving people the client has contact with uncertain about the effects of their actions on the client. Other clients may provide critical rather than constructive feedback. Constructive feedback emphasizes how the client feels or thinks about someone else's behavior that is experienced as aversive and emphasizes what might be done instead. The goal should be to tell the other person nonpunitively about the effects of his or her actions and clarify what could be done to achieve better outcomes. Constructive feedback provides descriptive rules, rather than punishment.

Making Requests for Behavior Change. Another repertoire closely associated with providing constructive feedback is making effective requests for change in others' behavior. There are two critical dimensions of effective requests.

1. Requests are different from demands. Many people, particularly in intimate relationships, make demands for immediate change in others' behavior. Such demands are generally experienced as aversive by the listener and are for that reason resisted. A request states or asks for what the person making the request would prefer (for example, "I would appreciate it if . . ." or "Could you . . .") rather than tells the other person what he or she must do ("You call me if you are going to be late coming home from work from now on!").

Clinical Practice with Individuals

2. The request must be specific and behavioral rather than general and vague. For example, "I would like to sit down together after dinner and see if we can make a plan about how to handle housekeeping" is much better than "I want you to start doing your part around here!" The first statement makes it clear what is desired (this is just the beginning of the process), whereas the second is vague and has a punitive edge that is likely to lead to conflict.

Being Nonprovocable. Reseach done with couples indicates that in nonconflicted relationships at least one partner is "nonprovocable" (Burman, John, & Margolin, 1992). *Nonprovocability* means that the person does not punish the other for doing something unpleasant. Reciprocation, in contrast, is likely to lead to an escalating coercive spiral. Nonprovocability is probably useful in a broad range of relationships. Not punishing someone does not mean reinforcing; some version of ignoring is involved in effective nonprovocable repertoires, and practice is required to do this effectively. Self-talk strategies also are often needed.

Refusing Requests and Demands. One important dimension of assertiveness is being able to effectively say no to unreasonable demands or requests or those that would result in unacceptable costs. Some clients passively agree to such requests even when the requests are unreasonable or inconvenient; others may be able to say no but find themselves becoming irritable and aggressive while doing so. Identifying specific ways to say no (including specific phrasing—for example, "I'm sorry, I can't do that now because . . .") and practicing how to do this in an assertive way (in which all parties are treated with respect) are often required.

Negotiating. Negotiating solutions to issues and conflicts requires the application of many important relationship skills, including recognizing and respecting everyone's rights and interests, listening actively and empathically, making specific requests and suggestions, refusing unacceptable solutions but proposing reasonable alternatives, and providing both positive and constructive feedback. Problem-solving negotiation can be conceptualized as consisting of four steps: (1) identification of the issue, (2) clarification of each person's understanding of and interests in the issue, (3) identification of possible options, and (4) evaluation of potential consequences of each option—ultimately leading to a decision. This process is similar to choices and consequences (presented in previous chapters) but makes provision for involvement of each of the individuals with an interest in the issue.

Skills Training Techniques

Only a few of the skills described in the previous section can reasonably be the focus of clinical work at one time, and those listed, although widely applicable, are certainly not exhaustive. Decisions about where to focus should be made as part of an individualized assessment of each case. Once skill deficits have been identified, several common behavioral strategies are useful for teaching the selected repertoires, including instructions, modeling, rehearsal, feedback, work with self-talk, and homework. In most cases, some mix of these techniques is required.

Instructions. Simply providing instructions can be a good beginning for teaching new repertoires, particularly when the rules for effectiveness are clear. Teaching clients to make "I" statements, maintain eye contact, or speak a bit louder are examples. Instructions, however, often produce only a first approximation of effective behaviors, and additional techniques are usually required to shape adequate repertoires. In addition, behavior that is primarily or excessively rule bound may not be as sensitive to changing circumstances (variations in antecedents and consequences) as that shaped by direct contingencies through the use of modeling, rehearsal, and feedback.

Modeling. In modeling, the social worker demonstrates one or several possible options that might produce better outcomes in situations with which the client is struggling, and the worker and client then collaboratively refine effective responses. Other people also can be used as models; for example, the clinician may ask a coworker who is similar to the client or is effective in particular areas to step into the session and model while the worker and client take the roles of others in the social scene of interest. The worker and client also may begin with the behavior of someone not present; for example, the worker can ask the client how a respected television character or someone the client knows and respects would respond to the social situations faced by the client (refer to "Fixed-Role Therapy" in chapter 3 [pp. 52–53] for more information).

Rehearsal. Rehearsal is graduated practice in social scenes analogous to those that are difficult for the client. It is a form of role playing with a special problem-solving purpose. As such, rehearsals should be as realistic as possible. In most cases, the worker begins by either providing instructions for or modeling the desired response. The client is then asked to try the approach. The most straightforward way to use modeling and rehearsal is for the clinician to model interacting with the client first and then to switch roles. Other possibilities are available, including speaking to an empty chair (adapting a Gestalt therapy technique) or bringing one or more additional people into the session. For example, a male social worker may have a male client who does not have the skills to ask a woman out but wishes to. The scenario may seem realistic if, after a female coworker of the social worker comes into the room, the clinician models appropriate dialogue, and the client then imitates the modeled actions. (This approach also offers opportunities to use contingent feedback; see below.)

Several specific techniques can make rehearsal more effective. If the client begins by saying, "Well, I would say that I wanted . . ." the worker should gently interrupt and model the actual statement: "I want . . ." (it is important that the client actually practice not just describe). The worker also can quietly prompt the client, providing fragmentary modeling as the client is rehearsing, and gradually fade the prompts:

Social worker   (taking role of friend the client would like to ask to go to a movie): Yo, Sam, what's up?
Sam: Not much.
Social worker: Cool.
(pause)
Social worker   (in quiet voice, pointing toward client): What are you doing . . .
Sam: What are you doing tonight?
Social worker: Good! Let's try it again. . . . Yo, Sam, what's up?

The worker using this technique needs to be sure to differentiate clearly between when he or she is the role and when he or she is prompting and reinforcing Sam; this is easy in practice (by using a different, quieter voice or giving physical signals). Similar prompting can be used in situations in which a third party has been brought into the room to take a role.

The form of rehearsal described above because of its similarity to real-life cues is widely applicable in clinical work. Another variety of rehearsal, *covert rehearsal*, is useful in situations in which realistic stimulus conditions are difficult to replicate in the session. In covert rehearsal, clients are asked to imagine (often after closing their eyes) the challenging situation, then to talk their way sequentially through the interaction, as if running a movie in their imaginations. At the appropriate points, the client vocalizes the dialogue ("He says . . .; then I say . . ."). The social worker can prompt and reinforce throughout this process. Covert rehearsal is a useful skill for clients to learn, because they can apply it on their own to prepare for future challenging social encounters.

Contingent Feedback. Feedback lets clients know how effectively they are using new repertoires. Such feedback should be framed in a positive way that leaves room for improvement. For example, a first awkward attempt could be reinforced with, "That's a good start! This time, you might try . . . ." If the next effort is an improvement, the worker might say, "Better! You're getting there. Try once more; maybe you also can try looking at me when you say it this time." If the second attempt is not better, the worker can simply say, "Not quite. Let's try again." Humor can often reduce tension in this process and communicates that it is not critical that the client perform perfectly right away (or in fact ever).

Some workers question whether it is better to keep providing specific instructions for improvement during this process (for example, about exactly what to say or how to say it) or simply to give global feedback for each effort (for example, "That's better" or "Not quite" or "That's about a 5 on a scale of 1 to 10"). Specific feedback may simplify the process by adding a layer of rule governance, but some evidence suggests that global feedback may sometimes result in more effective behavior (Hayes, Kohlenberg, & Melancon, 1989).

Self-Talk. Changing self-talk has been discussed extensively in previous chapters. Some clients will report, if asked, that they tend to carry on a running dialogue with themselves while they are trying to handle difficult situations. This dialogue may distract and interfere with performance, and it is important for clients to develop ways to interrupt their self-talk and focus exclusively on what the other person is saying. Others may find the self-talk (and relaxation) strategies presented in the discussion of inoculation procedures in chapter 5 helpful, particularly in preparing for and entering potentially anxiety-producing social situations.

Homework. Clients want to learn new social repertoires so they can handle situations in their lives more effectively, not so they can be more effective in discussions with the social worker. Therefore, clients should practice new skills in everyday interactions when they begin to feel ready to do so. Homework tasks of several kinds can be useful here. Some challenging situations (such as opportunities to refuse unreasonable demands) may come up unexpectedly; after practice in the session, the client may take on an assignment to spend time with people who are likely to make such demands and to keep a log of what happened. The log should include what the other person demanded, how the client responded, what the results were, how the client felt, and what he or she was saying to himself or herself throughout the incident.

The client can initiate practice in other skills. Logs such as those described above or simple records of how many times the client made an effort can be kept of those attempts. A valuable self-monitoring technique is to count how many times one performs positive targeted behaviors on an ongoing basis. A client who decides to provide social reinforcers more richly to members of his or her family can carry an inexpensive golf stroke counter in a pocket and advance it each time he or she verbally compliments or expresses appreciation to a family member. (Pads and small pencils work well for many kinds of behavior, although they are slightly more obtrusive than the golf counters.)

Booster Sessions. Unless the natural environment richly reinforces clients' first efforts, new repertoires may fade before fluency is reached. In addition, clients' situations sometimes change and become more challenging. For these reasons, it is valuable to schedule one or more booster sessions some weeks after the completion of skills training to provide additional support and refine skills. These sessions can be planned, or the social worker can tell the client that this is an option. If the second approach is used, it is essential to clarify that deciding to return for a booster session is not a sign of failure but rather a recognition by the client that more work may make him or her stronger and better able to face difficult challenges.

USING SKILLS ON APPROPRIATE OCCASIONS

Many people have skills that they do not use when they might be effective, and they often use less than optimal parts of their social repertoires. Many people who become verbally abusive and punitive with family members act more respectfully with their employers; respectful behavior is in their repertoires, but a problem exists with stimulus control. Under these circumstances, clinical intervention aims to help clients learn to use the right skills at the right time. Two basic approaches are useful here: (1) becoming aware of differential occasions and (2) experimenting by using available repertoires under different conditions. Some clients also benefit from learning how to behave in ways that more effectively set the tone for the occasion and motivate others to be responsive to them.

Discriminating among Occasions

Behavior is often learned under circumstances and maintained by factors of which the client is unaware (in traditional terms, the reasons for the behavior are unconscious). An awareness of the circumstances that evoke ineffective social behavior and of appropriate circumstances for applying existing or recently learned skills is valuable for clients. Clients are then in a position to provide self-instructions (rules) for themselves; for example, "If I ask my partner to do me a favor when she is under a lot of stress, she will probably get angry, and we may have a fight. If I wait until the pressure is off, she will probably happily agree." Timing is everything in social relations.

Identifying appropriate occasions for using social skills is important. During the right circumstances, saying "I love you very much" will lead to deepening intimacy. On other occasions (too early in a relationship or with a person in an inappropriate role) the same behavior may have negative consequences. Similarly, self-disclosure may be appropriate on some occasions and not on others. For example, a client had a granddaughter who was born after an incestuous relationship between the client's two teenage children. This disclosure in clinical work was important, but the client habitually discussed her granddaughter's history with most people she met, including school staff members, other parents at the child's school, and even people with whom she had routine business dealings. Helping to discriminate appropriate occasions for self-disclosure is an important interventive goal for this and similar clients.

Sometimes cultural and cohort differences make it confusing to identify which social behavior will be effective in a situation. Members of certain Asian cultures make extensive use of indirect communication, whereas members of many American Indian cultures particularly respect directness. Many people who grew up and developed social skills in the 1960s and early 1970s tend to be more affectionate verbally and physically with friends than are members of some older and younger cohorts. Even the cultures within particular families

Clinical Practice with Individuals

vary widely. Not surprisingly, many clients struggle to respond in appropriate ways on different occasions.

Many clients, when they are under pressure, strike out figuratively or literally at others. (The stressful conditions—motivating antecedents—increase sensitivity to aggression reinforcers.) The goal of intervention may be to reduce aggression. Two nonexclusive alternatives are available for doing so. First, the worker can help the client discover ways to reduce the stress. Second, the clinician can help the client learn that stressful times are occasions for being particularly careful to act in sensitive ways to those around them. Assuming the new behavior works and is reinforced, the client may then be more likely to continue to act in this sensitive way under pressure.

Several strategies exist for learning to discriminate occasions when one behavior will be effective from those when another will produce better results. Sometimes, the social worker or people in the environment with whom the client can inquire can provide straightforward instructions that the client can learn to follow. A second strategy is for the client to observe others who effectively discriminate among occasions to determine what they do and when. The client may then be able to learn by imitation. Finally, the client may need to experiment and to try acting in different ways (which can be developed in the clinical session) and determine inductively what the results are.

Implementing Skills Differentially

Experimentation can help extract effective rules for effective social behavior. The value of experimenting, however, goes beyond this. It is one thing to be able to describe verbally how to act at particular times but another to do so effectively. Many people who are members of couples are verbally abusive to their partners, even though they know this is undesirable and do not want to continue doing so. Knowing what not to do, however, is not adequate; undesirable behavior is likely to continue despite self-punishment until the client has other alternatives available.

Those other alternatives often must be functionally equivalent to the problem behaviors. Irritation and aggression toward a spouse during work-related stress may be one way to avoid further pressure and demands. On the same occasion (when the spouse makes a request) and under similar contextual conditions, such clients need to practice different repertoires (for example, a respectful, assertive refusal) that will also provide relief from the perceived demands. Only by practicing alternative responses (often first rehearsing in session, then perhaps rehearsing with the partner, and only then under actual life conditions) are clients likely to experience the differential consequences that will maintain the new repertoires. Homework assignments are particularly important here because they provide opportunities to experience better payoffs from alternative social acts.

Providing Occasions and Motivation for Others to Relate to the Client

Many clients need to learn how to act differentially in ways likely to work well for them on differing occasions, and many also need to learn how to act so as to make it more likely others will behave well toward them. As an example, clients with poor personal hygiene may drive others away (the way someone looks and smells can be a motivating antecedent for escape by others). More subtle conditions also are commonly involved, however. People who constantly complain about their lives and the people around them often find themselves increasingly isolated. Other people have learned that spending time with people who act like that seldom produces reinforcing consequences.

Clients can do many things to prepare for social interaction with other people, including dressing well, paying attention to personal care, beginning conversations in pleasant ways, and using humor. Many clients have skills that can make them rewarding social partners but need to use them on the right occasions. One of my clients, a bright but socially isolated graduate student, had a particularly creative, dry humor. When discussing current events, his view of them was often extremely entertaining, but he had gradually stopped reading the newspapers. When he started to read them again and practiced ways to start conversations about what he read, he became an engaging conversational partner to whom others responded. As a result, he experienced an increase in positive social attention.

SOCIAL NETWORK SUPPORT SKILLS

As with any other behavior, new social skills are shaped and refined and will be maintained only by consequences in the client's life. Ensuring that clients are exposed to situations that will reinforce new repertoires is crucial. No aspect of assisting clients who are experiencing relationship and social difficulties is more important than working to increase exposure to new sources of social reinforcement. In social work, if a client returns to the same toxic environment that shaped earlier failures, in most cases the old problems will re-emerge. Occasionally, a client will quickly develop new skills to connect with social networks in the old environment that were previously not accessible without explicit help, but this is not common. A major focus of intervention often must be assisting clients to obtain access to social networks that will reinforce newly learned skills.

Identifying or Constructing Networks

Clients who have been isolated for a long time often are at a loss as to where to find friends. If their skills are also limited, not all social environments are likely to be tolerant enough to allow them to participate before their repertoires are adequately honed. Helping the client to identify multiple options, including family, friend, work, church, school, and socialization groups; recreational or political organizations; and volunteer opportunities, is useful. This identification can be challenging, because many clients have had so many bad experiences that they may at first seem resistant to even discussing such options. If that happens, the social worker may want to clearly separate discussion of possibilities from commitments to pursue them; this approach can sometimes reduce anxiety considerably. Many possibilities are open to each client, but it may take substantial collaborative work to identify them and to explore how the client might achieve them. Although it can be frustrating to help a client investigate several possibilities only to ultimately reject them, experience suggests that eventually the client will identify a network that appeals to him or her if the worker simply keeps reinforcing efforts and does not punish the client for hesitating.

The worker also can take steps to change the networks within which the client is embedded (as in family therapy or in meeting once or twice with a friend or family member who might be willing to accompany the client on early social forays). In other cases, the worker may want to consider initiating some form of group service for these clients; the service could be something as structured as a socialization group or could be an alternative such as a social club focused on exploring restaurants or museums.

Experimenting

Once clients have learned new skills and have identified multiple settings and arrangements in which they can test them, the next step is to experiment in everyday life. This is a challenging step, and the worker and client should plan such experiments in small steps and with an expectation that not all will pay off right away (these are experiments, after all). Clients are likely to require considerable support from the worker to take the necessary steps and may find it helpful to take them in the company of someone with whom they are comfortable. Many clients find it helpful to collaboratively develop detailed possible plans but want to make the decision about when to implement the more challenging plans. Encouraging the client to take major steps too quickly is a mistake (although small ones are fine) because the client who fails to follow through—if doing so is more difficult than expected—may hesitate to return to the clinician and acknowledge failure.

It is also valuable for the social worker to normalize the struggles and let the client know that some experiments may not work. If the client recognizes that many possible experiments can be tried, no single one will become so important that a failure will be seen as a major setback. Helping the client to view the process as a sort of serious"play" and as something that will probably take time before results occur (rather like the way antidepressant medication takes time to begin to work) may be helpful in reducing pressure. Work with relationship problems can involve a focus on one but more often on two or three key dimensions: learning the skills; assisting clients to use skills on occasions in which they are likely to be effective; and assisting clients to expose themselves to social networks that will reinforce initial attempts, even inept ones, to practice social repertoires.

VIOLENCE IN RELATIONSHIPS

An especially troubling problem in intimate relationships is physical violence, which is an extreme form of social coercion. Battering is a serious social issue, and social workers in any setting need to have complete familiarity with recognition of battering and with intervention for both victims and perpetrators. Several points are worth noting here. First, violence is behavior; as behavior, it is shaped by its consequences. Violence is not caused by triggers, it is not caused by mental illness, and it is not caused by substance abuse, although these antecedents may have some influence. Violence occurs because it works (even though it may be costly as well). Violence can have multiple functions—some violence occurs because it reduces aversive stimulation and other violence occurs because it produces positive reinforcers (for example, money) (Mattaini, Twyman, Chin, & Nam, 1996).

Battering occurs because it results, at least sometimes and up to a point, in control of the other person—it is at root a deeply coercive act (see Mattaini, Twyman, Chin, & Nam, 1996; Pence & Paymar, 1993). Like other coercive acts, violence produces negative consequences for everyone involved. These negative consequences, however, are delayed, whereas the power and control achieved are immediate. Viewed in this way, clearly the goal for the batterer must be to bring his or her behavior under the control of rules (for example, "No matter how angry I get, I am responsible for my actions" or "If I feel myself becoming very angry, I must leave the situation and cool off") rather than immediate, direct-acting contingencies. He or she (it is usually, but not always, a man, and battering also occurs in gay and lesbian relationships) must also learn that no one has the right to hit another person in an intimate adult relationship. If the partner's behavior is truly unacceptable, the other has the choice to make a strong request for change or to leave but never to coerce. These are also rules, the unstated part of which is that if he or she handles the situation in a way other than through violence, he or she and others will ultimately experience a much better outcome.

The person who is battered is not at fault. In many cases, social workers can help victims to problem solve (choices and consequences) and to deal with the depression and demoralization resulting from the abuse; much of the discussion in previous chapters is relevant here in terms of helping the victim or survivor to feel and act in an empowered way. At the same time, it is critical to reinforce the client both for considering and for taking positive steps without punishing, even subtly, if the client is not ready to do so. Many women return to the men who have battered them. Although this act may be undesirable from the worker's perspective, the decision can be understood based on financial, emotional, and even safety considerations (women who leave their batterers are at exceptionally high risk during the early stages of separation). It is the worker's responsibility to respect the woman's right to make her own decision, clearly advocating that she do what seems best to her but helping her to carefully examine alternatives. Support groups have been demonstrated to be particularly helpful under these circumstances (Tutty, Bidgood, & Rothery, 1993).

The goal for the batterer is also clear: To relate to this or any future partner with respect for his or her equality and right to make his or her own decisions. Requesting and providing sincere appreciation for what is desirable is fine, but demands, coercion, and punishment in adult partner relationships are never acceptable. Little is known about how to help batterers move toward this stance despite many—sometimes conflicting—strong opinions (Fagan & Browne, 1993). There is some evidence that group interventions can be effective, although most voluntary participants drop out of such groups early. Couples work is generally not indicated, because it may put the victim at increased risk.

Batterers who are voluntary clients often are seen individually. Within an ecobehavioral model, several possibly effective interventive strategies emerge. Substantial focus on learning new rules and bringing behavior under the control of those rules is essential. A first step is to assist the person to accept that battering is not acceptable under any circumstances (although this is purely anecdotal, my clinical experience suggests that men who engage in clinical consultation voluntarily are sometimes close to accepting this fact, although involuntary clients are often far from doing so). Choices and consequences, with particular emphasis on planning strategies that will lead to safety, is crucial. Anger inoculation (see chapter 5) may well be useful, and planning and rehearsing specific steps the client can take at high-risk moments (for example, putting on his coat, leaving, and staying somewhere else) might make it much easier to take that step later. Rehearsal and practicing of alternative ways to relate to the partner also may be helpful using self-monitoring and self-management strategies. Ideally, the partner also should be concurrently involved in his or her own consultation focused on safety and empowerment strategies. These directions are based on clinical experience and theory but have not been empirically tested. Still, they may provide some beginning strategic directions when working with individual voluntary clients involved in intimate violence.

REFERENCES

Burman, B., John, R. S., & Margolin, G. (1992). Observed patterns of conflict in violent, nonviolent, and nondistressed couples. *Behavioral Assessment, 14,* 15–37.

Carnegie, D. (1981). *How to win friends and influence people.* New York: Pocket Books. (Original work published 1936)

Fagan, J., & Browne, A. (1993). Violence between spouses and intimates: Physical aggression between women and men in intimate relationships. In A. J. Reiss, Jr., & J. A. Roth (Eds.), *Understanding and preventing violence: Vol. 3. Social influences* (pp. 115–292). Washington, DC: National Academy Press.

Follette, W. C., Bach, P. A., & Follette, V. M. (1993). A behavior-analytic view of psychological health. *Behavior Analyst, 16,* 303–316.

Gordon, T. (1970). *Parent effectiveness training.* New York: Wyden.

Hayes, S. C., Kohlenberg, B. S., & Melancon, S. M. (1989). Avoiding and altering rule-control as a strategy of clinical intervention. In S. C. Hayes (Ed.), *Rule-governed behavior: Cognition, contingencies, and instructional control* (pp. 359–385). New York: Plenum Press.

Lowery, C. T. (in press). Hearing the messages: Integrating Pueblo philosophy into academic life. *Journal of American Indian Education.*

Mattaini, M. A., Twyman, J. S., Chin, W., & Nam, K. (1996). Youth violence. In M. A. Mattaini & B. A. Thyer (Eds.), *Finding solutions to social problems: Behavioral strategies for change* (pp. 75–111). Washington, DC: APA Books.

Pence, E., & Paymar, M. (1993). *Education groups for men who batter: The Duluth model.* New York: Springer.

Rakos, R. F. (1991). *Assertive behavior: Theory, research, and training.* New York: Routledge & Kegan Paul.

Stuart, R. B. (1980). *Helping couples change: A social learning approach to marital therapy.* New York: Guilford Press.

Tutty, L. M., Bidgood, B. A., & Rothery, M. A. (1993). Support groups for battered women: Research on their efficacy. *Journal of Family Violence, 8,* 325–343.

CHAPTER NINE

ADDICTIVE BEHAVIORS

E very social worker has clients who are involved with substance abuse or who have other problem behaviors that are commonly labeled "addictive" (although many such cases are commonly missed by clinicians). However, the severity of genuine addictions should not be trivialized by calling everything an addiction. In this chapter, the term addiction is used for patterns of behavior that appear to involve substantial changes in physiological responses, including alcohol and drug abuse, some eating disorders, and uncontrolled gambling, all of which can lead to severe life consequences. (So-called addictions to "love" or "dysfunctional relationships" are primarily relationship problems; see chapter 8.) The primary emphasis in this chapter is on problems related to alcohol and drugs (legal and illegal) given the high rates of these problems experienced by clients seen by social workers and the severity of those problems. Many of the principles, however, can be usefully applied to help people troubled by other addictive behaviors.

About 5 percent of American adults experience severe dependence on alcohol at any one time, but perhaps one-fourth of the adult population has some level of problems related to alcohol use (Sobell & Sobell, 1993). If family members, employers, and others indirectly affected are counted, the number is substantially higher. Approximately 15 percent of Americans ages 12 and older report the use of illegal substances each year, although not all of these people experience significant life problems as a result. Substance abuse is high among people experiencing some other forms of serious life problems, including violence, severe mental illness, and homelessness; causal relations among these issues are often reciprocal. For example, homeless people are often severely depressed and may turn to substance use for relief, but substance abuse contributes to both depression and homelessness. Problems related to addictive behaviors are widespread and costly to society and people, particularly social work clients.

The material in this chapter is not designed to be a complete elaboration of treatment for addictions, which is a specialized field. The intention is to present several straightforward ecobehavioral approaches for use by social work clinicians in general practice settings in which the primary focus is not on substance abuse but in which clients nonetheless experience these problems. The first section summarizes recent work in motivational interviewing, a collaborative approach for helping clients decide whether they wish to take steps to address problems resulting from substance use. This summary is followed by a discussion of assessment of addictive patterns. In many cases it is not the person using substances but those around him or her (family and employers in particular) who first recognize the problem. The unilateral family therapy approach, presented in the third section, and variations of it can be helpful under those conditions. A summary of a contemporary model of behavioral treatment for problem drinkers follows. This short-term, structured approach can be applied in many social work practice settings without major programmatic shifts. Finally, the community reinforcement approach (CRA), which is broadly applicable to work with addictions and is probably the contemporary approach that has so far produced the strongest empirical results, is outlined. Components of this approach can easily be integrated into community-based programs and can produce often surprisingly strong results.

As with other problems, ecobehavioral work with people struggling with addictive behaviors should be viewed as collaborative consultation rather than as a confrontational and coercive process. The first stance is more respectful and more likely to be effective. The second may lead to resistance and denial, is likely to fail, and places the clinician in a potentially untenable role. Even in involuntary settings, the real work does not begin until the client is ready to acknowledge and collaborate on solutions to the problem. In some cases, it may be valuable for others in the client's social network to present their views of the consequences of the abuser's behavior and of the further consequences that will follow if changes are not made. Even under those circumstances, the decision to act must be the client's.

MOTIVATIONAL INTERVIEWING

The first step in changing any addictive behavior is for the client to determine that he or she has concerns about use of substances. An emerging strategy for being helpful in this stage is motivational interviewing, developed by William R. Miller and his colleagues (Miller & Rollnick, 1991). Motivational interviewing is an alternative to confrontational approaches, which often elicit denial rather than a commitment to change, and is consistent with common European practice in substance abuse. The core notion is to collaboratively assess, with the client, patterns of substance use and concerns about it, moving finally toward identifying active steps to address the issues surfaced. The worker avoids telling the client what to do or insisting that the client has a problem and instead helps the client to explore and discover these things on his or her own.

Although motivational interviewing is commonly used in specialized substance abuse settings, the greatest potential for application may be in general practice settings, including many family services, health services, and other agencies in which social workers practice. (The following section closely follows Rollnick & Bell, 1991, pp. 203–213.) Experts in motivational interviewing suggest that it is important first to build rapport with the client and to establish oneself as a concerned and nonpunitive person. The next challenge is to raise the issue of substance use in a less confrontive way than, for example, by noting, "You obviously have a drinking problem!" Rather than beginning with substance use, the clinician should ask about general areas of concern that may be linked to substance abuse and through open-ended questions assist the client to explore these areas. At an appropriate time, the worker may then find it useful to inquire, "How is your use of alcohol connected here? Can you tell me a bit about that?" Questions such as these should be asked sincerely ; the client is the expert on his or her own life, whereas the worker's role is to assist the client to elaborate connections.

Rollnick and Bell (1991) offered several motivational interviewing strategies for use by the nonspecialist in general practice settings:

- In the course of the interview, explore the use of substances in a detailed way, primarily through open-ended questions, rather than simply asking whether the person uses alcohol and drugs (or worse, not asking at all). Useful questions may include, "Tell me about your use of . . .," and "How does alcohol affect you?"
- Ask about typical episodes in detail (for example, "So, you went to the bar right after work, and had . . . six? . . . drinks. How did it feel to have the first one?")

- Discuss aversive conditions and events the client deals with and how he or she copes with these. Substance use often comes up in such discussions of potentially motivating antecedents.
- Ask about substance use in the context of general questions regarding health and draw out connections.
- Ask about both what is satisfying about substance use (the reinforcers it offers—often called "good things" about use in motivational interviewing) and what is aversive ("less good things"). It is important, as in many other areas, to acknowledge that a behavior may produce multiple consequences, both positive and negative. Discussion of aversive consequences can lead to discussion of concerns.
- Ask about changes in substance use over time.
- Offer information and then ask about its application to the client. For example, the worker might provide basic information about increasing tolerance in a factual way and then ask, "I wonder if that applies to you?"
- Ask about the client's concerns. This is the central strategy toward which all of the others can move discussion. Once the client acknowledges use and some problems related to it, asking, "What concerns do you have about this?" will usually move the conversation a step closer to commitment to change.

The last strategy (eliciting concerns) is key; the others may be useful in moving in that direction. The worker would not ordinarily use all of these in a session; rather those that are appropriate to the client's situation can be mixed and phased.

Once concerns have surfaced, the worker should ask the client what his or her next step might be: "So, you're concerned about the health risks you are taking . . . What steps could you take next?" This is a challenging moment for both client and social worker. It is important that this step not be handled as a confrontation but rather as a move toward a basic problem-solving strategy such as choices and consequences (see chapter 4).

The motivational strategy outlined above can be applied to essentially any addictive behavior pattern. Once recognition of a possible problem has surfaced, it is important to understand it in further detail, particularly if the worker is going to work with the client around the issue or needs to determine what the best possible referral might be. The following section sketches a basic framework for such an assessment.

ASSESSING ADDICTIVE BEHAVIORS

In some cases, clients will come to the social worker acknowledging a problem with substance use and the clinician can assist the client to examine and understand his or her current pattern of use and the kinds of changes that could help. In other cases, the possibility of substance abuse may begin to emerge during discussions of other issues. Both types of situations call for the skills of motivational interviewing, although the worker may be able to move more quickly into an assessment of addictive patterns in the former. Information regarding the extent of use, physiological involvement, broader connections with other life spheres, and a functional analysis of substance use behaviors is needed to develop a collaborative plan with the client.

Use Patterns and Extent of Problem

Well-established protocols and instruments can be helpful in establishing the extent of substance use and related problems. For example, the four-question screening tool shown in Figure 9-1 (a recent modification of the CAGE screening protocol, which inquired whether the client has ever tried to *cut down*, ever been *annoyed* because someone complained about the client's drinking, ever felt *guilty* about drinking, and ever taken an *eye-opener*—a drink first thing in the morning) has proved reliable in identifying people in general

---

1. Have you thought you should cut down on your drinking of alcohol?

                    Yes   No

2. Has anyone complained about your drinking?

                    Yes   No

3. Have you felt guilty or upset about your drinking?

                    Yes   No

4. Was there ever a single day in which you had five or more drinks of beer, wine, or liquor?

                    Yes   No

Figure 9-1. A simple instrument to assess the possible presence of alcohol abuse. Excerpted from PRIME-MD™. © 1996. Reprinted with permission of U.S. Pharmaceuticals Group of Pfizer, Inc.

Clinical Practice with Individuals

medical settings who have alcohol problems (Mayfield, McLeod, & Hall, 1974; U.S. Pharmaceuticals Group of Pfizer, 1996).

If a client answers one question positively, the possibility of an alcohol problem should be explored; if more than one question is answered positively, the probability of a problem is high. With minor adjustments, similar questions may be of value in screening for other addictive problems, although the reliability and validity of this screening approach has only been established with alcohol.

Standardized instruments also may be useful, in particular for making a basic screening decision about the presence or absence of a possible problem (MacNeil, 1991; Seltzer, 1971). Such instruments and the four simple questions shown in Figure 9-1 have proved reliable and valid with general clinical populations; however, information collected under duress may be less accurate, because the contingencies involved are different. As with most other problems discussed thus far, not all substance abuse problems are the same; how, when, and under what conditions an individual client uses substances and the circumstances surrounding use are often crucial data for assessment. Self-monitoring can be a valuable way of obtaining such data and also may act as a motivating antecedent, increasing motivation for change.

Self-Monitoring. Several approaches to self-monitoring can be useful in working with addictive behaviors. It is critical to track the frequency of the behavior itself; in addition, monitoring urges or cravings and environmental conditions under which use or craving occurs also can be valuable. As is the case with standardized instruments and questionnaires, self-monitoring of the use of substances by clients has proved accurate (Sobell & Sobell, 1993). Self-monitoring can increase client motivation for change and also can facilitate empowerment (Kopp, 1993); observing the connections between behavior and other variables suggests to clients that if they can act to change those variables, they may thereby achieve an important level of self-control.

One approach to such monitoring is the time line follow-back method (Sobell & Sobell, 1993), a retrospective approach in which the client is asked to reconstruct the frequency of substance use during an extended period (for example, 90 days). The developers of the approach and their colleagues have demonstrated that the technique provides accurate data. Some clients may be able to complete the time line as a homework assignment using a blank calendar; in other cases, the worker and client may wish to collaborate. If the worker and client then identify and discuss patterns that appear to be present, important assessment information is likely to emerge. In this process, it may be important to examine the use of multiple substances; polydrug abuse is common among social work clients and may not be revealed unless it is specifically discussed.

Although information about use (or craving) is important, it is also crucial to identify the surrounding circumstances, because these are critical in conducting the functional analysis required for interventive planning. Instruments and standard forms are available for tracking these conditions and events (Miller & Muñoz, 1982; Sobell & Sobell, 1993); the best approach, however, may be for the clinician to familiarize himself or herself with these standard models and then to collaborate with the client to develop a variation that feels not too burdensome but captures the needed information. Some variation of a log capturing the time and place, potential triggers, people present, emotional and other situational factors, and the outcome of use or craving situations is useful; this log may consist of a narrative, a simple grid, or some other format. What is essential is that the approach used capture antecedents and consequences that may be important in developing an interventive plan.

Physical Dependence and Medical Status

Physiological involvement, including withdrawal and tolerance and associated medical conditions, often must be considered in work with addictions, in particular addictions to substances. Although physiological issues can to some extent be assessed verbally (for example, symptoms experienced in previous episodes of withdrawing from narcotics or increased tolerance with alcohol), complete medical examinations also should be arranged. In some cases, medical findings may clarify appropriate treatment goals (for example, a person with liver pathology should probably not consider a controlled drinking goal—see "Working with Clients Involved in Problem Drinking" on pp. 155–157 for discussion of the controlled drinking controversy) as well as interventive strategies. Withdrawal from some substances can be life-threatening; the social worker is ethically bound, therefore, to know to what extent this is true for the chemicals being used by the client and to ensure that necessary medical referrals are made.

Ecobehavioral Scan

As with any serious human problem, addictive behaviors are determined by many factors and embedded in complex contextual situations. For example, people with few positives in life are at high risk for addiction to crack cocaine (Leukefeld, Miller, & Hays, 1996; Mattaini, 1991). Environmental conditions, events, and people provide important consequences related to substance abuse beyond those provided by the substance itself (for example, a client whose primary social network revolves around a neighborhood bar), and they also may provide a range of important antecedents (for example, places and people that may become associated with substance use [occasions], models, and motivating antecedents).

Identifying high-risk situations or triggers—people, places, circumstances, and emotional factors—that come to be associated with substance use is a major consideration in the treatment strategy called *relapse prevention* (Marlatt & Gordon, 1985). Within this approach, clients are warned about the abstinence violation effect (for example, people who use drugs for the first time after a period of abstinence may think that all their hard work is lost and then continue into a full relapse). This effect need not happen, however. Relapse prevention emphasizes developing coping strategies for individually identified high-risk situations and presents relapses as interruptible opportunities for learning rather than as total failures.

Theoretical advantages exist to separate those antecedents that become occasions for substance use (for example, bars) from those that increase sensitivity to the reinforcers resulting from use (motivating antecedents). Places, times of day, companions, activities, or most anything else can come to be occasions for drinking or drug use simply through repeated temporal association. For most people with addictions, limiting exposure to such situations and learning coping strategies for circumstances when they cannot be avoided are important repertoires to strengthen.

Other people may model the use of alcohol and drugs, may provide rules ("you'll like this" or "everyone cool uses this"), and may reinforce use and punish refusal. It is common for substance abusers to be embedded in cultures of drug and alcohol use. Participation in such cultures goes well beyond stimulus control (occasions) and may need to be interrupted for an adequate outcome. A lone drinker may be helped by becoming immersed in a richer social network, but a client who is part of a drug-using subculture may need to leave that group and connect to alternative networks that will reinforce a sober, drug-free lifestyle.

Finally, the relapse prevention literature suggests that negative emotional states are commonly associated with some relapses to substance use, and the matching law also suggests that a person who experiences substantial deprivation (few reinforcers) and high levels of aversives is likely to be particularly sensitive to the biological and perhaps social reinforcers resulting from substance use. (Most drugs of abuse provide physiological reinforcement; for example, by mimicking the effects of natural endorphins.) This fact may be far more clinically significant than it first appears. For example, for a young person of color, a lifetime of oppression and pain associated with racism may be a powerful motivating antecedent for any behavior that provides even temporary relief from anger and demoralization. Learning new strategies for coping with these experiences may be effective, but discovering ways to actively change such contextual factors may be even more important. The latter strategy involves empowerment; genuine empowerment requires involvement in a network in which the coercive power modeled by the dominant society is rejected in favor of the sharing of power, a complex but critical repertoire (Lowery, in press; Lowery & Mattaini, 1996).

Functional Analysis

The early stages of assessment for substance use involve collecting data regarding the frequency of substance use, associated social and medical problems, and the ecobehavioral situation within which substances are used. Once this information has been gathered, the clinician and client are ready to tentatively identify the functions of substance use for the individual involved. All cases are not alike, and such an analysis may be important in planning.

For example, a young woman who drinks far more than she wants to when she is extremely anxious in social situations is likely to require a different interventive strategy than a client experiencing severe depression who drinks continuously or another who drinks when another person treats him or her badly. Although occasions, rules, and models are important to consider, an adequate functional analysis for substance use should focus particularly on identifying motivating antecedents and consequences associated with the addictive behavior by an individual client. Once these have been identified, active collaborative plans to change the conditions and consequences experienced by the client become the core of intervention.

PROGRAMMED REQUESTS FOR CHANGE IN ADDICTIVE BEHAVIORS

Traditional wisdom in substance abuse treatment suggests that a person with an addiction problem needs to be ready for change and those around him or her need to learn "loving detachment." The data suggest that this view is not only oversimplified, it is sometimes simply wrong. It is clear from research and clinical experience that those around the substance abuser sometimes enable the addictive behavior, for example, by covering for the abuser at work or in other ways preventing the abuser from experiencing the natural consequences of his or her behavior. (Note that suggesting that people sometimes fall into enabling patterns as a result of environmental contingencies does not mean they have a disorder called *codependence*. This label, which has little or no empirical support, unfortunately has often been used as a way of placing responsibility for others' problems on women; Anderson, 1994.) Practically all professionals working with family and significant others of substance abusers now recommend that those people stop performing those behaviors that enable the abuse.

In recent research conducted by Edwin J. Thomas and his colleagues, it has become clear that, in some cases, the people most significant to substance abusers can affect other contingencies related to the abuse (Thomas & Yoshioka, 1989; Thomas, Santa, Bronson, & Oyserman, 1987). Before describing their program, however, several clarifications are in order.

First, social workers should make it clear to the client that suggesting that significant others can have an impact on substance use should not be read as stating that these people are to blame for the chemical abuse. Contingencies arranged by family can make a difference in the lives of children with developmental delays or people with diabetes, but this does not make the family responsible for the problem.

A second crucial point is that only under certain (sometimes unclear) circumstances do family and others have enough control of the relevant contingencies to influence the substance abuser. The program discussed here can be helpful in maximizing this influence, but when this proves inadequate, the client is best referred to an Alanon group to learn loving detachment and acceptance (which sometimes in the long run also influence the substance abuser by changing social antecedents and consequences associated with substance use).

If the social worker's client is the spouse, partner, or another highly significant person in the life of a substance abuser and a collaborative decision is made that one goal of consultation is to arrange contingencies that maximize the client's influence on the behavior of the substance abuser, Thomas's program, which he calls *unilateral family therapy,* may be of particular value (Thomas, Santa, Bronson, & Oyserman, 1987; Thomas & Yoshioka, 1989). The program was developed specifically for this purpose, although aspects of it have broad applicability in many other relationship issues. Unilateral family therapy has much in common with the "interventions" that are now often arranged for substance abusers, in which a network of family, friends, employers, and whoever else is affected by the substance abuse confronts the user and attempts to induce him or her to enter treatment. Unilateral family therapy differs, however, in that it directly applies behavioral principles and can be effectively used when only one person (usually the partner) is available. The following paragraphs, assume that the client is the partner of the substance abuser, but in other cases it may be, for example, a parent. The material in this section provides an introduction to this approach; the worker who plans to use it should refer also to the original sources.

In unilateral family therapy, consultation revolves around three areas: (1) assisting the partner to enrich his or her own life (using any of the other strategies presented in this book), (2) working with the partner to change the contingencies in which substance use is embedded, and (3) asking the abuser to change in the most effective way possible.

Enriching the Partner's Life. Thomas and his group (Thomas et al., 1987) discovered in their research population that the first area did not usually require extensive attention, but this may not be the case in typical agency settings. If in the course of clinical assessment the client determines that an effort to influence the addictive behavior of a significant other should be among the goals, unilateral family therapy provides a well-explicated way to pursue this.

Changing Contingencies Involved in Substance Abuse. Five strategies are used in this phase of unilateral family therapy (the last three strategies all involve direct changes in the contingencies in which the abuser is embedded):

1. The partner monitors the use of the substance to further determine the extent of the problem.

2. Alcohol education is provided as needed.

3. The partner provides a higher level of reinforcers for the abuser (at times when he or she is not abusing substances) on a temporary basis to improve the relationship and potentiate the partner as a source of reinforcement. The partner as a source of reinforcement is important at a later stage when the partner requests change.

4. Most partners have previously attempted to change the abuser's behavior through punishment and other coercive acts. The fourth core strategy is to neutralize the previous influence system—essentially, to discontinue these ineffective efforts, which also increases sensitivity to the programmed request for change made later.

5. The partner discontinues behaviors (for example, buying alcohol, covering up, or drinking with the abuser) that reinforce substance use and protect the abuser from the natural consequences of his or her behavior (disenabling).

Requesting Change in Substance-Using Behavior. Once the partner has made whatever changes are possible, the stage is set for the next phase: requesting change. Thomas and his colleagues (Thomas et al., 1987; Thomas & Yoshioka, 1989) distinguish between a "programmed confrontation" and a "programmed request." Both involve a planned meeting between the partner and the abuser, usually with the clinician present and often but not always in the clinician's office. The difference between the two is that in a programmed confrontation the partner clarifies that, if the abuser does not immediately enter treatment, become abstinent, or both, the partner is prepared to carry out a serious consequence (for example, separation, divorce, or leading separate lives within the relationship); in the programmed request, the partner makes a carefully rehearsed request for change but does not indicate that he or she will carry out a consequence. The programmed confrontation option, in which the partner indicates he or she will take action if the abuser's behavior does not change, should be used only when the partner is ready to follow through on the consequences identified. If the partner is not actually willing to take specific, immediate action, the "programmed request" option should be selected; making an empty threat can be worse than doing nothing at all.

Both alternatives are forms of requests, but the programmed confrontation adds a description of future changes that will occur if the abuser does not take action. In both cases, the final choice is the abuser's. The ideal confrontation probably involves not so much a coercive threat as a clear description of the certain effects of continued abuse. The difference between making a coercive threat and providing a rule in this way is subtle but real. The partner is not saying, "I demand you stop now, or I will leave" but rather, "If you do not stop now, I will be unable to continue to live with you."

The nine steps involved in the programmed confrontation or request are shown in Figure 9-2. The basic strategy is for the partner, in collaboration with the social worker, to develop and rehearse a script to be used in the confrontation. Rehearsal prepares the partner to remain calm, not be distracted by defensive reactions, and deal with likely responses on the part of the partner. The overall tone of the confrontation is caring and serious, and arrangements should already have been made for the abuser to follow through on what is requested (for example, the partner can provide a phone number for a treatment program that has an immediate opening available).

---

1. Determination of suitability of situation for the unilateral approach

2. Determination of feasibility of spouse making programmed request

3. Preparation of spouse's script:
   a. Declaration of affection
   b. Statement of concern about drinking and its effects
   c. Specification of drinking level and severity
   d. Itemization of drinking-related incidents, problems, and their effects
   e. Specification of action recommendations
   f. Specification of consequences if action is not taken

4. Rehearsal of script

5. Staging of confrontation

6. Postconfrontation planning

7. Conduct of the confrontation

8. Postconfrontation monitoring and follow-through

9. Stabilization and maintenance

Figure 9-2. The steps involved in developing a programmed confrontation. Adapted with permission from Thomas, E. J. (1989). Unilateral family therapy to reach the uncooperative alcohol abuser. In B. A. Thyer (Ed.), *Behavioral family therapy* (pp. 191–208). Springfield, IL: Charles C Thomas.

Clinical Practice with Individuals

Rehearsal also should prepare the partner for "bargaining"; for example, some abusers will indicate that they will not enter treatment but will reduce their intake. The partner should think through the options and be prepared to make his or her minimum request clear. (See discussion later in this chapter about moderation as a treatment goal; for now, it is important to note that available data suggest this is a reasonable goal for some people but certainly not for all.)

For what clients might unilateral family therapy be appropriate? Research has focused on couples in which the partner did not have a substance abuse problem, in which there is no violence present, in which there is no serious active mental disorder, and in which alcohol was the only substance being abused. In clinical practice, some clients may need to make requests for changes in addictive behaviors even if not all of these criteria are met. The clinician should be sensitive to possible risks in such cases. In cases in which the partner also has a substance abuse problem, the partner's problem should usually be dealt with first. In cases in which battering is present, the violence should be the initial focus of treatment (see chapter 8), although substance abuse treatment may often be part of the intervention plan.

WORKING WITH CLIENTS INVOLVED IN "PROBLEM DRINKING"

Current data suggest that there are about four times as many people who might be classified as "problem drinkers" as there are people who are severely dependent on alcohol (Institute of Medicine, 1990). In recent years, attention has been focused on the former, who often can be effectively treated in nonintensive outpatient programs. In some cases, advantages exist in catching substance abuse early before more serious problems develop (note that the traditional belief that alcohol problems are always progressive has not stood up to empirical scrutiny). Certainly, pain and many personal, family, and other problems can be prevented if effective intervention with problem drinkers is available.

Social workers interested in consulting with this population should certainly read the available treatment manual (Sobell & Sobell, 1993), but a brief summary of the guided self-change treatment approach will be presented here. This approach is a structured outpatient model in which consultation consists of an assessment and four treatment sessions (there is room for flexibility in terms of number and frequency of sessions). The guided self-change approach is a self-management approach in which the clinician acts as a guide and consultant but in which the client does the bulk of the work.

In the guided self-change model, clients choose the goal toward which they will work, either abstinence or moderate (controlled) drinking. Despite ongoing controversy in the field, some problem drinkers, unlike most people with severe dependence, can do well with a goal of moderation. The issue is not as stark as it may seem; even strong advocates of abstinence often indicate that clients may need to try to achieve moderation before they are ready to recognize that that will not work for them. Note that moderate drinking as used here refers to controlled drinking, in which the person commits to particular limits and ways of drinking, not to uncontrolled social drinking. (In general, the recommendation is that the client's goal be no more than three standard drinks on no more than four days per week.) A moderation goal has yet to be tested with substances other than alcohol, although clearly some people use various drugs and do not become dependent. Practice wisdom in the field suggests a moderation goal is not realistic with other drugs (perhaps in part because of the illegal cultures within which use occurs), and until more research is done, the responsible course is probably to let clients know that.

Outcomes reported for the guided self-change approach are positive, producing major reductions in drinking and accompanying improvements in other areas of life functioning (Sobell & Sobell, 1993). Much of the work in the approach is done by the client outside the sessions, including completing readings and questionnaires. For clients with minimal literacy, adjustments have to be made. The following is the basic outline of the approach.

Assessment. During the assessment, clients are screened to determine whether guided self-change treatment is a reasonable model for them; clients also are asked to provide data in a number of areas, including a time line follow-back drinking history, an inventory of drinking situations (used for functional analysis), and a goal statement. Clients are breath-tested for alcohol use and provided with forms for monitoring consumption, a short reading, and a written homework assignment to complete before the first treatment session.

Session 1. In the first treatment session, the clinician and client review the self-monitoring logs; review the first reading (which relates to antecedents and consequences of drinking); and discuss answers to the first homework assignment, which prompts the client to complete his or her functional analysis of drinking. Material on relapse prevention also is covered in the reading and discussion; although research on the model has not yet supported the need for this focus, the developers believe it may be valuable and have found eliminating it somewhat awkward. The importance of completing the program is emphasized.

Session 2. Before this session, the client has completed a lifestyle assessment checklist, which is useful in thinking about changes in how the client spends his or her time, where, and with whom, that may be important for achieving the goal. The client and social worker review this assignment, along with the self-monitoring logs and material covered in the first session.

Session 3. The third consultation focuses on problem solving, particularly around ways to deal with high-risk situations. Before the session, the client has completed a reading assignment covering developing action plans (similar to choices and consequences as used in this book) and completed written action plans for his or her highest risk situations. As in every session, logs are reviewed and the importance of completing the program is emphasized.

Session 4. In this final formal session, the client completes a new goal statement based on what has been learned during treatment, and the worker and client discuss the homework assignments completed for the earlier sessions. This session consists largely of review and consolidation. Plans for follow-up contact are clarified.

It may be necessary to modify this straightforward program for specific clients; one of its particular advantages is its emphasis on flexibility and individualizing within a broad structure. This model may have broad applicability within practice settings, particularly if it is used within an ecobehavioral perspective that takes all relevant factors of the client's life situation into account and within which problem drinking may be one significant issue.

COMMUNITY REINFORCEMENT

Each of the approaches discussed so far in this chapter can be used by an adequately informed and trained worker in any clinical setting. The final ecobehavioral model is CRA, which is probably best provided in a specialized treatment program, but because CRA programs are not widely available and given persuasive data for the efficacy of the approach, clinical social workers should probably be prepared to adapt it for use in other settings.

CRA has demonstrated impressive effectiveness at modest cost in work with alcohol abusers and cocaine abusers and appears promising for work with other addictive behaviors (Meyers & Smith, 1995). In one study with inpatient alcohol abusers, at the six-month follow-up session, clients receiving standard treatment (alcohol education, 12-step counseling, and encouragement to be involved in Alcoholics Anonymous and to take Antabuse) were drinking on 55 percent of days, whereas the CRA group averaged drinking on 2 percent of days (Azrin, 1976). In an outpatient study, the CRA group was abstinent on 97 percent of days, whereas the standard treatment group averaged abstinence on 45 percent of days (Azrin, Sisson, Meyers, & Godley, 1982). In one of several studies involving cocaine abuse, only 5 percent of subjects dropped out of the CRA program after one session compared with 42 percent in the traditional treatment group; 58 percent of the CRA group completed the full 24 sessions compared with 11 percent of the comparison group. Sixty-eight percent of the CRA group achieved eight continuous weeks of abstinence, whereas only 11 percent of the traditional group did so. These results (and those of other studies of the CRA, all of which are consistent with these) are far from perfect but are impressive for substance abuse treatment programs.

Reinforcement Networks

CRA is an outstanding example of an ecobehavioral approach to understanding and helping with serious clinical problems. The approach involves a mix of multiple components (summarized below), but it is the entire system (Meyers & Smith, 1995) that is crucial. The core of CRA is helping the client to establish an alternative network of consequences and antecedents that ensures that sober and drug-free behavior is more rewarding than drinking or drug use. The behavioral ecomaps shown in Figures 9-3 and 9-4 demonstrate this concept. The left panel in Figure 9-3 depicts contingencies associated with drinking for Client A, whereas the panel on the right shows the few existing supports for behavior associated with sobriety.

Figure 9-4, by contrast, shows the goal state for Client A: a richer arrangement of reinforcers and different antecedents, all supporting sobriety. The purpose of CRA is to build this sort of alternative overall network of

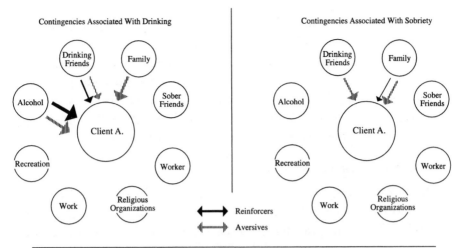

Figure 9-3. Behavioral ecomaps contrasting contingencies associated with drinking and those associated with maintaining sobriety.

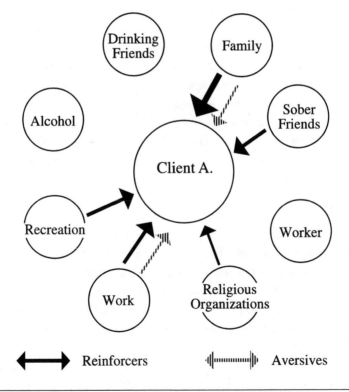

Figure 9-4. A reasonable goal state for the client shown in Figure 9-3.

community reinforcement for the client. Specific components of CRA are designed and selected to help establish such an arrangement. Some are essential for most clients, especially strong social support from concerned others (for example, spouses); a stable, sober, and drug-free friendship network; and a reinforcing job that does not put the client at risk for substance use. Support from all major dimensions of the client's life (work, family, and friends) is marshaled in the CRA to maintain an alternative lifestyle.

Contingency Management Procedures

In work with drugs other than alcohol, contingency management has been added to the standard CRA components in several studies and appears to be useful. The general procedure has been a system in which clients can earn vouchers that can be used to purchase prosocial items or participate in activities (for example, movie tickets, recreation equipment, or restaurant certificates) for clean urine samples. These arrangements often include a program of accelerating rewards, in which longer drug-free periods produce higher daily payoffs. Although this program involves some costs ($12.36 per day in one study but tapered to two $1.00 lottery tickets per week after 12 weeks of more intensive treatment; Budney, Higgins, Delaney, Kent, & Bickel, 1991), these are short-term costs and are modest compared with the expense of inpatient treatment. Some creativity may be required in agency practice to make provision for such immediate reinforcers, and they may need to be included in agency budgets. In one project with which I am involved, a program for homeless substance abusers offers incentives such as tokens for public transit, small cash bonuses, and access to special food donations for increasing periods of clean urine samples.

Components

In assisting the client to develop habits that reinforce a sober and drug-free lifestyle, the developers of CRA have tested and refined multiple discrete components, which are summarized here. It is important while examining these components not to view the list as a sort of á la carte menu, from which those that are most easily addressed are selected, but rather to maintain focus on achieving a rich, multidimensional network of reinforcers for this new, alternative lifestyle. Some of the skills-training components—for example, drink refusal and assertiveness—are means to an end. The overall need for a new, richly fulfilling lifestyle is the goal of the approach and must be kept firmly in sight.

Clinical Practice with Individuals

Functional Analysis. The functions of substance use are explored in CRA to determine not only antecedents that may place the client at risk but especially the consequences that may be supporting use. Refer to the section "Functional Analysis" under "Assessing Addictive Behaviors" earlier in this chapter for further information.

Reciprocal Relationship Counseling. Concerned significant others, particularly spouses, partners, and other family members, are among the most crucial sources of important social contingencies for many people. Building levels of positive exchange, reducing levels of aversive exchange, and improving communication are often important aspects of constructing a rewarding, sober life. The experience of the developers of CRA has been that brief intervention focused on increasing positive reciprocity is useful.

Job Counseling and the Job-Finding Club. A fulfilling vocational arrangement (usually involving a job or school) is important for everyone, including those striving to recover from addictions. In CRA, every effort is made to assist the client to obtain and maintain a vocational situation that is rewarding and does not set the client up for relapse. For example, many clients with serious alcohol problems should not work in bars. Those who have previously used drugs when on their own for long periods should work in a setting that involves considerable contact with others rather than in an isolated position such as a night guard at a warehouse.

Community reinforcement approach programs have often established job-finding clubs, formal group arrangements in which clients assist each other in looking for jobs, preparing application materials, and preparing for interviews. Although a clinician working with one or a few substance-abusing clients may not have the population required to establish such a club, in agency settings there are often many clients experiencing a variety of problems (not just substance abuse) who might benefit from such a club. Outcome data for job-finding clubs are promising, and social workers interested in establishing them should refer to Azrin, Flores, and Kaplan (1975).

Social and Leisure Counseling. Satisfying lives usually involve more than love and work; opportunities to play also are important. Many substance-abusing clients have limited repertoires in this area or may have discontinued involvement in leisure, recreational, and social activities. It is important to emphasize this life sphere by helping clients think about options, assisting them to learn to access those options, and encouraging them to sample those they have never experienced or have not experienced for many years. (Such reinforcer sampling can be a powerful motivating operation, increasing sensitivity to new reinforcers.) Because some clients lack social and communication skills necessary to achieve satisfying social relationships, social skills training may be required. Training in general problem-solving and assertive repertoires are often needed. Community reinforcement approach programs often establish alcohol-free social clubs to give clients access to social activities and mutual social reinforcement without placing them at risk. Buddy systems in which a client is connected with someone who will help in maintaining sobriety in part by assisting the client to be active in social and leisure activities are yet another useful approach.

Antabuse Assurance. Antabuse (disulfiram) is a medication that a person takes to assist him or her to remain sober. If a person taking an adequate dose of Antabuse drinks any alcohol, he or she will become ill (people taking it have to carefully avoid alcohol-based mouthwashes, aftershave lotions, and so forth). The medication generally produces only minimal if any side effects so long as the person remains alcohol-free. The research suggests (and this makes considerable theoretical sense) that simply providing a prescription for Antabuse usually results in noncompliance. The Antabuse assurance procedure—a standard component of CRA—embeds taking Antabuse into the client's social network and has proved effective. Each day the client asks a concerned other to provide the medication and takes it in the presence of the other person. In this way, taking the medication is initiated by the client, which is a different situation than if the concerned other demanded that the client take it. The client only needs to make a decision once a day about whether to drink while taking Antabuse and needs to wait for a couple of days after discontinuing Antabuse before drinking can be safely resumed. When used in CRA, the medication is generally taken to provide short-term assistance to avoid impulsive drinking for the first 90 days of sobriety (often a high-risk period). By this time, the client will usually have achieved a measure of stability in a new, sober lifestyle.

Early Warning Systems. Several variations of CRA include some form of early warning system in which the clinician is informed as quickly as possible about circumstances that may lead to a relapse. One component of the Antabuse assurance procedure is usually that the client or concerned other contacts the clinician if the client fails to take the medication two days in a row. When couples reciprocity counseling is part of the program, each member of the couple is often asked to complete a brief marital happiness scale and return it by mail every day for several weeks. Clients are commonly seen twice a week early in treatment.

Immediate feedback such as this appears to be helpful to many clients for whom impulse control is an issue. For example, I was seeing a client for a pattern of behavior that the client viewed, justifiably, as a sexual addiction. He struggled for several months to bring this problem under control before we hit on a procedure that ultimately proved effective. He would call my answering machine every night before going to bed to report on how he had done that day. If he missed more than one day, which only happened once or twice, I called him. This procedure, in which the client only needed to stay with his self-management program "one day at a time," seemed to have been a turning point for this young man.

Sobriety Sampling. In sobriety sampling, the client makes a contract with the clinician to remain sober for a brief period, perhaps one day or until the next session. Like the early warning system, it seems to be helpful for many clients to build a significant period of sober or drug-free experience day by day and seems to be helpful in building motivation and commitment over time.

Skills Training. Clients often feel uncomfortable saying no when others offer them drinks or drugs, particularly if the person offering pressures or embarrasses the client in any way. In refusal training, using standard social skills training procedures, the worker helps the client to construct and rehearse ways to refuse a drink or drugs. Many clients need to learn to say no in a simple but assertive way ("no, thank you"), more emphatic strategies for dealing with some kinds of pressure, and indirect approaches that are difficult to argue with ("No, thanks, my doctor says I need to avoid alcohol now"). Clients often need to have a range of such repertoires available from which they can choose depending on circumstances. Although the need to add relapse prevention training to the standard CRA procedures has not been clearly established, it is sometimes included in the package and may be of value to many clients. Relaxation training is sometimes included as an alternative coping strategy within relapse prevention.

Other Components. A number of other components are sometimes included in CRA, depending on the population served, and some may be important in social work cases. Substance abusers often have many other life issues to address (which can be identified by developing a behavioral ecomap with the client). Many clients require intensive and wide-ranging case management services, including advocacy to help them access needed services. In programs dealing with homeless clients, attention to basic needs, including housing, food, clean clothing, showers, and mail service, may need to be included. By taking a broad ecosystemic look at the client's life situation, the worker can begin to identify sources of aversives and deprivations of basic needs and reinforcers that may need to be addressed if the client is to construct a more reinforcing life.

Implementation: The Sharing of Power

Variations of CRA could be implemented in any social work setting where the necessary expertise regarding substance abuse is present. Several critical considerations exist in doing so.

First, the worker should pay consistent attention to the overall levels of reinforcers and aversives the client has available, not just details related to specific treatment techniques. If a sober, drug-free life is not adequately rewarding, the risk of relapse is high. Clients are unlikely to give up sure reinforcers associated with substance use if nothing is available to replace them.

Second, the model suggested here is heavily collaborative rather than confrontive, building on the motivational interviewing techniques discussed earlier. It is not the worker's job to coerce the client to become sober and drug free (and efforts to do so are unlikely to work). The social worker needs to work in concert with the client to share responsibility with the client for developing a plan that can work. Within the team of worker, client, and concerned other that may evolve, everyone has expertise, resources, and knowledge to contribute; only by working together can this team develop the power needed to overcome the control of strong contingencies that maintain addictive patterns. Shared power is constructive power (Lowery & Mattaini, 1996).

This last note reflects wisdom provided by American Indian cultures that is of potential value to everyone—one enormous advantage of cultural diversity is that insights learned and nurtured by one culture can be useful to others faced with difficult circumstances. Culturally specific strategies also can be important to the success of CRA and the reasons are clear: what is rein-forcing to a member of one culture (for example, attention and recognition) may not be reinforcing to a member of another—and may even be aversive. Clients and concerned others from the client's own culture are the experts regarding what kinds of important reinforcing networks need to be con-structed to assist a particular client in achieving and maintaining a sober, drug-free, and fulfilling life.

Addictive behaviors are, at base, behaviors. Although they involve a sig-nificant physiological component (including biological reinforcers and aver-sive physical conditions), the principles for changing these behaviors are the same as for any other. The client, clinician, and concerned others col-laborate to complete a functional analysis and understand the ecobehavioral contingencies within which the addictive behavior is embedded, then de-velop and implement a plan to change the contingencies and arrange access to alternative sources of reinforcers. Given the high personal and social costs of addictive behaviors and their substantial prevalence rates in the popula-tion, every social worker should be familiar with basic approaches such as those presented in this chapter for working with clients who are struggling with these issues.

REFERENCES

Anderson, S. C. (1994). A critical analysis of the concept of codependency. *Social Work, 39*, 677–685.

Azrin, N. H. (1976). Improvements in the community-reinforcement approach to alcoholism. *Behaviour Research and Therapy, 14*, 339–348.

Azrin, N. H., Flores, T., & Kaplan, S. J. (1975). Job-finding club: A group-assisted program for obtaining employment. *Behaviour Research and Therapy, 13*, 17–27.

Azrin, N. H., Sisson, R. W., Meyers, R., & Godley, M. (1982). Alcoholism treatment by disulfiram and community reinforcement therapy. *Journal of Behavior Therapy and Experimental Psychiatry, 13*, 105–112.

Budney, A. J., Higgins, S. T., Delaney, D. D., Kent, L., & Bickel, W. K. (1991). Contingent reinforcement of abstinence with individuals abusing cocaine and marijuana. *Journal of Applied Behavior Analysis, 24*, 657–665.

Institute of Medicine. (1990). *Broadening the base of treatment for alcohol problems.* Washington, DC: National Academy Press.

Kopp, J. (1993). Self-observation: An empowerment strategy in assessment. In J. B. Rauch (Ed.), *Assessment: A sourcebook for social work practice* (pp. 255–268). Milwaukee: Families International.

Leukefeld, C. G., Miller, T. W., & Hays, L. (1996). Drug abuse. In M. A. Mattaini & B. A. Thyer (Eds.), *Finding solutions to social problems: Behavioral strategies for change* (pp. 373–396). Washington, DC: APA Books.

Lowery, C. T. (in press). The sharing of power: Empowerment with Native American women. In L. Gutierrez & E. Lewis (Eds.), *Women and empowerment*. New York: Columbia University Press.

Lowery, C. T., & Mattaini, M. A. (1996). *The use of power in social work*. Unpublished manuscript.

MacNeil, G. (1991). A short-form scale to measure alcohol abuse. *Research on Social Work Practice, 1*, 68–75.

Marlatt, G. A., & Gordon, J. R. (Eds.). (1985). *Relapse prevention: Maintenance strategies in the treatment of addictive behaviors*. New York: Guilford Press.

Mattaini, M. A. (1991). Choosing weapons for the war on "crack": An operant analysis. *Research on Social Work Practice, 1*, 188–213.

Mayfield, D., McLeod, G., & Hall, P. (1974). The CAGE questionnaire: Validation of a new alcoholism screening instrument. *American Journal of Psychiatry, 131*, 1121–1123.

Meyers, R. J., & Smith, J. E. (1995). *Clinical guide to alcohol treatment: The community reinforcement approach*. New York: Guilford Press.

Miller, W. R., & Muñoz, R. F. (1982). *How to control your drinking*. Albuquerque: University of New Mexico Press.

Miller, W. R., & Rollnick, S. (Eds.). (1991). *Motivational interviewing: Preparing people to change addictive behavior*. New York: Guilford Press.

Rollnick, S., & Bell, A. (1991). Brief motivational interviewing for use by the nonspecialist. In W. R. Miller & S. Rollnick (Eds.), *Motivational interviewing: Preparing people to change addictive behavior* (pp. 203–213). New York: Guilford Press.

Seltzer, M. L. (1971). The Michigan Alcoholism Screening Test: The quest for a new diagnostic instrument. *American Journal of Psychiatry, 127*, 89–94.

Sobell, M. B., & Sobell, L. C. (1993). *Problem drinkers: Guided self-change treatment*. New York: Guilford Press.

Thomas, E. J. (1989). Unilateral family therapy to reach the uncooperative alcohol abuser. In B. A. Thyer (Ed.), *Behavioral family therapy* (pp. 191–208). Springfield, IL: Charles C Thomas.

Thomas, E. J., Santa, C., Bronson, D., & Oyserman, D. (1987). Unilateral family therapy with the spouses of alcoholics. *Journal of Social Service Research, 10*(2–4), 145–162.

Thomas, E. J., & Yoshioka, M. R. (1989). Spouse interventive confrontations in unilateral family therapy for alcohol abuse. *Social Casework, 70*, 340–347.

U.S. Pharmaceuticals Group of Pfizer, Inc. (1996). *PRIME-MD™*. New York: Author.

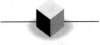

CHAPTER TEN

SEVERE MENTAL AND BEHAVIOR DISORDERS

S ocial workers often work with people who have severe mental illnesses and behavior disorders. Practice with these clients requires a mix of case management, education, and personal and family clinical consultation; none of these modalities by itself is likely to be adequate for this work. The discussion in this chapter applies, with variations as noted, to clients struggling with psychoses (including schizophrenia, schizoaffective disorder, and mood disorders of psychotic dimensions) and certain personality disorders involving severe and pervasive behavioral problems.

Although much is yet to be learned about such issues, we know more than we did a generation ago. For example, schizophrenia, which affects perhaps 1 percent of the adult population and usually emerges in late adolescence or early adulthood, clearly has biological roots. Schizophrenia is not the result of poor parenting or other life experiences, although given a biological propensity, life events (in particular, aversive factors) can play a part in the severity and topography of symptoms and relapses. Even less is known about other disorders producing psychotic symptoms, but evidence suggests that these too have biologic roots, although their presentation and course can be significantly affected by environmental events.

Although scientists may find some as yet unknown genetic connections that are involved in behavior patterns labeled "personality disorders," at present no data support this assertion, and a reasonable argument can be made that the primary determinants of these issues relate to learning history. The role of the social worker in mental health settings serving clients living with psychosis is not to "cure" the underlying disorder but rather to assist clients to live in a satisfying and fulfilling way—to assist and empower them to improve the quality of their lives, as they would with any other social work client. Social workers should aim not only to reduce symptoms, or even re-hospitalization, but also to ensure that the overall configuration of the client's life be as reinforcing as possible while minimizing the burden carried by others, particularly family. This chapter examines a number of discrete strategies (for example, medication, skills training, and family work) for work with people with serious mental illnesses. These strategies should be viewed as components that when properly mixed and phased can be valuable for assisting clients to construct reinforcing lives.

The social worker must see his or her function with all clients as joining the client and others in the social network in a collaborative effort to determine the desired outcomes and acceptable interventions. The power for change emerges from networks of mutual and noncoercive sharing and reinforcement. (Credit for conceptualizing effective practice as requiring the sharing of power in this way belongs to Christine T. Lowery, who has demonstrated the value of this traditional American Indian approach for social work practice; see Lowery, in press.) Unfortunately, it is common to slip into a coercive and often judgmental emphasis on compliance in cases involving severe mental illness. This emphasis may occur in part because client behavior that seems out of control may be aversive and frightening to the clinician and perhaps in part because placing people with mental illness in different equivalence classes from oneself may reduce the worker's own anxieties. Reminding oneself, therefore, that people living with mental illness are human and are often coping remarkably well with challenging biological, physical, and social conditions is particularly important.

MEETING BASIC NEEDS

Even before dealing with florid psychotic symptoms or severe family conflict, the worker must ensure that the client's basic needs are met. Many homeless people experience psychotic symptoms and severe depression and may perhaps be abusing substances as well (Rossi, 1989). Although many of the strategies in this and preceding chapters may be of use to these clients, unless structural antecedents that provide access to reinforcers (for example, health, food, or a stable living situation) and motivating antecedents (no more than manageable levels of deprivation) are in place, those interventions may not be of much benefit.

Conditions related to meeting client needs should not be artificially divided into separate categories (for example, concrete needs versus psychological needs). The client's environment and the contingencies that shape client behavior consist of a single field, and professional social work purpose involves work with this entire configuration. Although it may be possible in some cases to delegate efforts to meet certain needs to others, professional practice requires that the worker attend to all needs in some way. In ecobehavioral practice, the social worker's function is to empower the client to act in ways that result in obtaining adequate reinforcers (including tangible and social ones) and minimizing exposure to aversive factors; action to ensure that the necessary reinforcers are accessible is an organic part of this function. Whether the aversive situation involved is family conflict as a result of the client's bizarre talk or hunger resulting from deprivation, it should be included in the service plan.

A clinician's best behavior management skills may be required to arrange social and other contingencies in ways that make it most likely that collaterals (for example, family, agency representatives, or landlords) will act to make it possible for the client to have access to an adequate quality of life. The worker should not manipulate the client or use coercive tactics except when absolutely necessary; rather, adequate descriptions of why collateral action may be important (rules), constructive feedback, sincere appreciation, effective request making, advocacy, and the use of other interventive repertoires often call for the highest levels of professional expertise. When resources to meet basic needs are not available, the worker must sometimes help the client to accept the situation and achieve the best realistic adaptation, but this solution should always be recognized as undesirable and a reflection of the need for ongoing advocacy.

PSYCHOTROPIC MEDICATION

Many clients with severe mental illness need medication to manage their cognitive and emotional functioning; for many patients with schizophrenia, taking antipsychotic medications regularly minimizes the severity of symptoms and prevents full-scale relapses (Hogarty et al., 1986). Although the physician prescribes medications, the social worker has several important related functions. Remembering to take medication in the course of often disrupted and disorganized lives is difficult, and some patients find their medications unpleasant to take (although usually not as unpleasant as the symptoms that eventually emerge without them). Self-management techniques and regular monitoring may be valuable in these sorts of situations; the social worker often is in the best position to assist and reinforce the client for taking medications as prescribed.

The social worker also may need to provide ongoing guidance about how to take medication and why, because a client whose cognitive functions are disrupted may require more than a single explanation. Because antipsychotic and other psychotropic medications (such as lithium for bipolar disorders) are powerful drugs, it is important for everyone involved with the patient, including the social worker, to be familiar with and watchful for possible iatrogenic side effects (negative effects resulting from treatment). The worker also can often assist the client to manage active symptoms as well as possible; this assistance can be helpful in minimizing the required dosage of medication and possible side effects. Social workers in mental health settings should become familiar with the use of psychotropic drugs through coursework, supervision and continuing education, and reading (Bentley & Walsh, 1996).

PSYCHOEDUCATION

Although the term *psychoeducation* has come to be used broadly and sometimes inappropriately, it originated in work to teach people with schizophrenia and their families the facts about the disorder and how to live with it in as effective a way as possible. Many patients and their families know little about mental illness and often have substantial misconceptions. For example, parents who know little about schizophrenia often blame themselves for the occurrence of the illness in their children or blame the patient for his or her symptoms. These reactions often result in exacerbating the problems within the family. Education about the causes and symptoms of mental illness, medication, and how to live most effectively with the conditions can make a substantial difference. Studies consistently demonstrate that a combination of regular medication and family psychoeducation results in substantial decreases in symptom severity and the need for rehospitalization. Excellent replicable programs, especially for use with multifamily groups, are available for this work (Anderson, Reiss, & Hogarty, 1986).

Education about mental illness and medication also can be of particular benefit to clients themselves. Accepting a diagnosis of mental illness is not, however, an easy step for many people, and maximum clinical sensitivity is required to help the client through this process. Many clients associate mental illness with severe stigma (Link, 1987) and have formed equivalence relations such as

mental illness ≈ "crazy" ≈ social rejection ≈ hopeless

and therefore experience associating themselves with those relations as aversive. The worker's role in this case is to assist in changing these equivalence relations and the related self-talk. The reality of mental illness also involves substantial losses of actual or potential reinforcers (social, vocational, and other) for the patient and the family. These losses are another source of pain with which the worker must empathize while trying to build acceptance and hope that a fulfilling life can be constructed—or reconstructed. Not all clients are able to accept their diagnoses, particularly because cognitive functioning is, by definition, disrupted in many people with psychotic disorders. Even for those who cannot accept the diagnosis, education about specific areas (medication or family functioning, for example) may be of use.

MANAGING SYMPTOMS

A great deal of empirical evidence exists that bizarre speech and behavior for many people with psychosis can in part be shaped by environmental contingencies (Wong, 1996). The illnesses are not behavioral in nature, nor does the origin of symptoms lie exclusively in environmental contingencies. Rather, people with severe mental illnesses often have few repertoires available that produce significant natural or social rewards, making the behaviors they do have available likely to be emitted at high rates. Clients with psychosis often have few social skills that result in positive attention from those around them and, given the resulting level of deprivation, may emit bizarre behaviors that gain a significant amount of attention. As in many other areas, functional analysis is important, because topographically similar behaviors (those that appear alike superficially) may produce different consequences for different clients or under different conditions. For example, the function of bizarre talk for one client may be to obtain social attention, whereas similar behavior on the part of another client may result in escape from unpleasant social interactions.

The frequency of delusional speech can no doubt be increased if those around the person reinforce it richly, given a high level of social deprivation. It is also clear that high levels of bizarre talk tend over time to increase withdrawal by others (who usually find such talk aversive); this withdrawal may in turn result in escalation of the behavior. However, the answer is not simply to ignore bizarre talk, although one must be careful about reinforcing behavior likely to result in long-term isolation for the client. Helping the client to learn new, more socially acceptable ways to connect with others is critical; social skills are among the most important areas for skills training with this client group. Providing other ways to obtain valued reinforcers, concurrent with reducing reinforcement for undesirable actions (which result in poor long-term outcomes for the client), is likely to be effective. Learning a variety of skills that provide access to alternative forms of reinforcement is demonstrably effective in reducing the whole range of bizarre behaviors—see the section, "Skills Training," later in this chapter, for further detail.

Clients also are often disturbed by their symptoms, for example, if they hear voices (auditory hallucinations) or experience periods of derealization (when they feel out of touch with reality) or depersonalization (feeling out of touch with themselves). Sensitive clinical responses to these experiences sometimes require the worker to walk a fine line between reinforcing behavior that may be costly to the client over the long term (for example, extended discussions of the details of hallucinations) and assisting the client to cope with genuinely troubling symptoms. No single technique is available for doing so, but several clinical repertoires are valuable. One such repertoire is to empathize with the client's emotional experience rather than pursue the hallucinatory or delusional material itself (saying, for example, "It must be terrifying when you have that experience; can you tell me more about how you felt when that happened?").

A second critical clinical skill is to help the client re-examine for himself or herself the reality of delusional beliefs through a shaping process involving "tactful suggestions and leading questions" (Wong, 1996, p. 323). This re-examination includes work with self-talk (cognitive treatment) such as asking clients to consider alternatives or examining the evidence for the belief. Many clients eventually come to distinguish psychotic symptoms from reality ("It seems real, but I know it's not"). Supporting and reinforcing clients in making such discriminations can sometimes be helpful in minimizing the extent of medication required. This repertoire also makes it possible for some clients to avoid talking about symptoms in situations in which such talk may result in ostracism or social punishment.

SKILLS TRAINING

Many people with severe mental illness miss opportunities to learn a variety of life and social skills and commonly lose some of those they have previously learned. Skills training has been demonstrated to be an effective modality for reducing rehospitalization in addition to improving the client's quality of life (Hogarty et al., 1986; Wallace & Liberman, 1985). Training in functional skills, including work, social, and recreational skills, also can produce dramatic decreases in bizarre or repetitive behavior (Wong, 1996); given access to other, perhaps higher quality, sources of reinforcement, less behavior is allocated to the more limited alternatives.

Several categories of skills training, including social skills, self-care and independent living skills, vocational skills, and recreational skills, are often used with clients living with serious mental illness; each is briefly discussed below (see Wong, 1996, for a review). The basic technologies of skills training as discussed in chapter 5 are applicable with this population as well, including instructions, modeling, and shaping. The pace of training should be adjusted to the individual, and careful task analysis in which the overall task is broken into small pieces that can be learned and shaped sequentially is important. It is possible to begin with the last steps (for example, the last assembly task in some vocational training) and then gradually teach earlier and earlier steps (backward chaining) or to begin with the first steps and gradually work toward the goal (forward chaining). Generalization from training (for example, in social skills) in the office to other settings is often challenging for more regressed clients, and they may need a program explicitly designed with prompts and reinforcers provided in the natural setting. Because a certain level of skill may be required before natural reinforcers can maintain the behavior, it may be necessary to arrange or provide high levels of social and other reinforcers in the earlier stages of training.

Social skills can be particularly important because many people with psychotic and other behavior disorders who lack these skills experience severe isolation and social rejection. Conversation skills (including nonverbal and verbal components) such as how to greet another person, how to ask questions that further the conversation, and how to give compliments are often important.

Another critical component of social skills for people in community settings is assertiveness. For example, one of my clients with schizophrenia was often preyed on by people with whom he was acquainted who would ask him for money and even stay for extended periods in his apartment. Both direct case manager intervention and teaching assertive behavior were required to resolve these issues. Many clients also experience high levels of frustration and may act aggressively out of self-protection. Learning assertive alternatives can be important in those cases; for example, if a client is feeling stressed and overstimulated (see "Work with Family Systems," next page), being able to ask for some personal space can prevent the initiation of an aggressive and coercive spiral that can damage relationships and in some cases lead to relapse.

Self-care and independent living skills, ranging from maintaining personal hygiene to cooking and nutrition to financial management, are essential to an adequate quality of life and are often vital for maintaining health and well-being. In addition, many of these repertoires are essential for adequate social functioning, because they may make clients (and their homes) more attractive and inviting. Some of these skills may be lost over the course of illness and some may never be learned, particularly for those whose prodromal symptoms began to appear at an early age. Self-management techniques (because some activities—for example, doing dishes—are not immediately reinforcing to many of us) and basic skills training strategies can be valuable in these areas.

Vocational activities produce crucial tangible and social reinforcers for people, and this is often true for people with mental illness as for anyone else, although pacing and capacity need to be considered. Clinical social workers may not be responsible for training in this area in most cases but often need to advocate to ensure that the client is connected to opportunities to learn the needed skills. The clinician also may work with the client to strengthen certain related repertoires, such as job search and interviewing skills and social skills required to maintain employment.

Recreation is an important source of enjoyment, socialization, and stimulation and can be valuable for reducing bizarre and other undesirable behaviors. Unfortunately, many clients with mental illness lack both the skills and opportunities to engage in such activities. Access to opportunities is discussed below; skills training in this area is much like the other areas discussed thus far, except that natural reinforcers may take over more quickly in this area than in many others.

WORK WITH FAMILY SYSTEMS

Work with families (or other caretakers) is outside the domain of this book. However, because families have substantial importance in the lives of most people with severe mental illness (nearly half of people with severe mental illness live at home and most others have continued contact with family), a brief discussion is warranted. In schizophrenia, although a genetic vulnerability must be present if the illness is to emerge, stress is clearly associated with the severity and probably the frequency of relapse. Certain kinds of aversive and intrusive family environments appear to be difficult for many people with schizophrenia to manage. Much of the research in this area has focused on *expressed emotion* in the family. Expressed emotion is an atheoretical construct that emerged inductively from research related to patients with schizophrenia. The measurement of expressed emotion consists of three scales scored from a structured interview: (1) criticisms by family members, (2) emotional overinvolvement, and (3) the presence or absence of hostility. Most but not all of the research done on expressed emotion suggests that patients from high expressed emotion families are at higher risk for relapse (Halford, 1991). Extrapolating from these findings, most professionals assume that similar processes in other living settings also may place clients at increased risk.

Substantial unevenness and lack of clarity are present in the expressed emotion research, which suggests that, although the construct is capturing something important, more complexity may be present than first appears. Recent work by Halford (1991) suggests that escalation of reciprocal coercive interactions is common in families with high expressed emotion. Similar patterns have been clearly established in the families of aggressive youths (Patterson, 1976) and in marital distress (Gottman & Levenson, 1988). Many disturbed families develop cultures of mutual coercion, and changing these patterns may be critical to providing a manageable living situation for many people with severe mental illness. Coercive cycles can develop in families as a result of the enormous strains placed on both the patient and other family members by the illness. Although some families may have serious problems in family functioning before the illness, many do not. In either case, changes often can be achieved through family psychoeducation and behavioral family intervention carried out in the home (Falloon, 1988).

Two significant and often interrelated problems in families who take on the heavy burdens of care for family members with severe mental illness are dealing with common "negative symptoms" of the illnesses such as apathy and lack of active involvement and dealing with conflicts within the family. Many people with severe mental illness demonstrate substantial social withdrawal and an apparent lack of interest in daily activities; many parents in particular are disturbed by the client's apparent laziness and do not recognize these behavior patterns as part of the illness. Education and work on acceptance by family members is important here, as is problem-solving negotiation and communication enhancement among everyone involved.

Family work must often proceed gently and noncoercively to keep the level of emotional arousal and stress on the person with mental illness as limited as possible. Family members also may benefit from learning about options for dealing with other disturbing symptoms (such as delusional talk and aggressive behavior) (refer to Reid, 1992, for further discussion). Social workers practicing with the families of people with severe mental illness should familiarize themselves with the extensive literature in this area (see the reference list at the end of this chapter for places to begin).

LIFESTYLE ENRICHMENT

Service systems often are set up to ensure that the physical and safety needs of people surviving with psychosis and other severe mental illnesses are met so that the level of aversive factors clients experience is manageable. Even clients in model programs, however, report limited satisfaction in other areas of life, including social interation; essentially, they have the skills and resources to access only a limited range of reinforcers. Working with the client to develop as rich a lifestyle as possible is an important dimension of practice. Although contact with the worker is one source of enrichment, a much deeper and broader network is usually required to reach a reasonable level of fulfillment.

Many possible sources of pleasure and social support may be available, but a good deal of creativity by worker and client may be required to discover what works for a particular client. General categories to consider include the following:

- recreational activities, including spectator activities such as music, movies, or watching sports; involvement with computerized electronic communities; and participation in clubs
- outdoor activities, which provide a different class of reinforcers than urban activities for many of us, whether done alone or with others

Clinical Practice with Individuals

- involvement in self-help groups, which have demonstrated an extraordinary capacity to empower many clients with severe mental disorders, providing social connections, prompts, and reinforcement for taking steps to manage their lives
- vocational activities at whatever level the client can manage, whether in a regular job, in assisted employment, or in a sheltered workshop setting
- volunteer work, which can provide a sense of belonging and of making a contribution
- involvement with religious groups, which are sometimes particularly tolerant of atypical behavior
- ethnic-cultural associations.

Some clients may have a clear idea about what they would like to do (often because they enjoyed those activities in the past) and can be helped to acquire and refine the repertoires to succeed in those activities. Many clients, however, can benefit from sampling multiple potential sources of reinforcers from which they can then select.

A critical factor in making such plans is to determine the client's capacity and interest for social interaction. For example, one woman with bipolar disorder I have seen episodically finds group activities stressful but does well with activities that expose her to other people to a limited extent, such as swimming and using a gym. Another young man found it was important for him to be around people every day (and found reading in a cafe satisfying) and to have some interaction without intense conversation (and so joined a wrestling group for gay men).

The specifics matter enormously, of course, but the social worker also should keep in mind the overall configuration of the client's life. Any major sources of unmanageable aversive factors must be addressed (by client, worker, family, agencies, collaterals, or some combination), and adequate and varied sources of truly valued reinforcers need to be present and accessible. Social workers should look at each client as the center of a dynamic, living ecomap and not be too distracted by details.

YOUNG ADULT CHRONIC CLIENTS

In recent years, social agencies have reported an increasing number of young adult clients presenting with multiple concurrent problems, often including severe mental illness, substance abuse, involvement with the criminal justice system, and pervasive problems in personal and social functioning (often regarded as symptomatic of personality disorders, but see below). Many of these clients (called "young adult chronic patients"; McLaughlin & Pepper, 1990, p. 137) experience frequent crises and can be difficult to engage and work with. Several crucial points are important to keep in mind about these clients:

- Their behaviors, although challenging for the social worker, are the result of learning history and biology and are in some way functional for the client; "blaming the victim" is no more appropriate with these clients than with any others.

- These clients generally experience the conditions in which they live as highly coercive and aversive, and the experience of many with caretakers and helping professionals has been negative. Their sometimes desperate attempts to make changes, given their deficits in crucial repertoires, often make things worse, and it is not surprising that they sometimes turn impulsively to sources of immediate gratification, such as drugs and alcohol.

- Because many have grown up under unpredictable conditions, providing some stability and constancy is often an important aspect of intervention, but this stability need not, and should not, be primarily punitive, even though some of these clients may frustrate the social worker.

One frequent issue for such clients is substance abuse. Because of the way that service systems and funding streams are organized, many clients with dual diagnoses (mental illness and chemical addiction) find it difficult to obtain access to services. People struggling with addictions often do not fit eligibility criteria for mental health programs, and substance abuse programs often prefer not to work with those with serious mental and behavioral disorders. Many of those programs also have policies refusing to permit the use of psychotropic medications that clients with psychotic or mood disorders may require. The social worker may need to advocate for the inclusion of these clients in service settings and may need to work actively to educate coworkers, family, and others who come into regular contact with the client about the issues the client faces (for example, about mental illness and substance abuse) and the uneven progress to be expected.

All of the approaches discussed in previous chapters for dealing with addictions and relationship problems are applicable to this population. In addition, the worker may need to keep in mind the need for consistency and the need to keep returning to contracting and motivational interviewing, because such clients often have lived lives of chaos in which working toward long-term goals was unknown. Progress, therefore, often requires a gradual and extensive shaping process. Particularly helpful are clear contracts around contingencies, as in incentive and "level" systems, often within a community reinforcement approach (see chapter 9). Such systems can provide a new experience of consistency and need not be punitive but rather should be structured to encourage success and gradual strengthening of rule-governed repertoires.

Many of these young clients have been diagnosed as having personality disorders, particularly borderline and narcissistic personality disorders or disorders of the self. From an ecobehavioral perspective, many difficulties can occur with such diagnoses both in terms of their reality and their clinical usefulness. Disorders of personality have been described as "pathologies of the entire person" (Davis & Millon, 1994, p. 43), certainly a serious and not hopeful characterization. As it happens, personality disorder diagnoses have proved difficult to establish reliably, in part because they have been defined heterogeneously (people with different mixes of symptoms can be given the same diagnoses; Kutchins & Kirk, 1986; Mattaini & Kirk, 1991). In addition, the notion of a stable entity called a "personality" is inconsistent with the data (Mischel, 1968, 1986). When examined carefully, behavior has proved to be sensitively responsive to situational factors.

If one begins with the assumption that the client's behavior is shaped by learning history and current conditions, the prognosis is more hopeful (Mattaini, 1994). Certainly, the behavior of many such clients has been over-learned and has been reinforced inconsistently (as a result, it is difficult to eliminate given this intermittent reinforcement). However, if the clinician begins with a view toward helping clients to develop and practice repertoires that will result in better quality and more consistent consequences from their environments, rather than in fixing hypothesized intrapersonal defects, much can be done.

Many young adult clients diagnosed with personality disorders also are said to have defects of the self. Excellent behavioral and cognitive–behavioral work have been done in this area in recent years. Kohlenberg and Tsai (1991) have traced the reasons why many such clients have an inconsistent experience of "I"—they have difficulty making clear discriminations, such as "I feel . . ." or "I want. . . ." Kohlenberg and Tsai hypothesized that this inconsistent experience occurs because of inconsistent consequences during early years for identifying feelings, desires, and experiences. For example, at some moments saying "I am frightened" during appropriate conditions may have been reinforced but at other times ignored or punished ("No, you are not frightened!"). If Kohlenberg and Tsai's hypothesis is correct, an important clinically relevant repertoire for such clients may be developing an ability to clearly state their experiences of what is aversive and what is reinforcing without punitive consequences.

Another issue with many such clients relates to overly rigid equivalence relations, as a result of which people and experiences are viewed as all good or all bad, without subtle gradations. For example, consider the differences between the relation

$$\text{angry person} \approx \text{bad person (under any conditions)}$$

and the alternative relation

$$\text{angry behavior} \approx$$
$$\text{unpleasant (under particular contextual conditions only).}$$

A change from the first to the second by means of the cognitive interventive strategies discussed in chapter 4 can make a significant difference in the client's experience. Small situational differences may also, for some clients, lead to rapid shifts from one rigid class to another (good to bad).

These phenomena have been extensively discussed by object-relations theorists from a psychodynamic perspective, using terms such as *splitting* and *idealization–devaluation*. The differences between the ecobehavioral and object-relations views are important, however. All of these phenomena can be viewed as being behavioral in nature, not the results of hypothesized intrapsychic structures that cannot be tested. These behavior patterns are rooted in and potentially responsive to changes in contingencies like any other behavior. Although changing these patterns is challenging given their reinforcement history, there is no empirical or theoretical reason to assume that they, like any other behavior, cannot be changed.

An increasing amount of information about work with young adult clients with chronic mental illness is becoming available (see contributions in section III of Cohen, 1990). Some descriptions of this population and interventive approaches for working with them have a decidedly judgmental and pejorative slant, failing to recognize that these clients, like everyone else, are doing the best they can given the repertoires and resources they have available. Because their experiences and sometimes their mental illnesses often interfere with the engagement process, they present as resistant. It is easy to understand how they could be viewed as difficult and why clinicians may prefer not to work with them. A change in the social worker's perspective, however, can in part remediate this difficulty.

In summary, the social worker's responsibility—with these clients as with every other group discussed in this book—is to assist the clients to access adequate high-quality reinforcers and minimize contact with aversive conditions and events. For those clients with access to few resources, this can be difficult. Practice occurs within the matrix of modern society, must be respectful of the client's experiences, must be concerned with changes in the behavioral field and the contingencies in which antecedents, behavior, and consequences participate. For members of oppressed and exploited groups who are constantly exposed to coercive abuses of power, including people of color, those with serious mental and physical disabilities, gay men and lesbians, women, and elderly people, connecting with richer contingency matrices can be significantly more difficult. Nevertheless, the mission of social work is to empower and assist clients to improve the conditions of their lives, not to repair their pathologies. This is, perhaps, a different view of clinical social work. It is not just "therapy," nor is its primary purpose to change the client's behavior. Clinical social work practice is about improving clients' transactions with their worlds in ways consistent with the well-being of the community.

REFERENCES

Anderson, C. M., Reiss, D. J., & Hogarty, G. (1986). *Schizophrenia and the family*. New York: Guilford Press.

Bentley, K. J., & Walsh, J. (1996). *The social worker and psychotropic medication: Toward effective collaboration with mental health clients, families, and providers*. Pacific Grove, CA: Brooks/Cole.

Cohen, N. L. (Ed.). (1990). *Psychiatry takes to the streets*. New York: Guilford Press.

Davis, R. D., & Millon, T. (1994). Can personalities be disordered? Yes! In S. A. Kirk & S. D. Einbinder (Eds.), *Controversial issues in mental health* (pp. 40–47). Boston: Allyn & Bacon.

Falloon, I.R.H. (Ed.). (1988). *Handbook of behavioral family therapy.* New York: Guilford Press.

Gottman, J. M., & Levenson, R. W. (1988). The social psychophysiology of marriage. In P. Noller & M. A. Fitzpatrick (Eds.), *Perspectives on marital interaction* (pp. 182–200). Philadelphia: Multilingual Matters.

Halford, W. K. (1991). Beyond expressed emotion: Behavioral assessment of family interaction associated with the course of schizophrenia. *Behavioral Assessment, 13,* 99–123.

Hogarty, G. E., Anderson, C. M., Reiss, D. J., Komblith, S. J., Greenwald, D. P., Javna, C. D., & Madonia, M. J. (1986). Family psychoeducation, social skills training, and maintenance chemotherapy in the aftercare treatment of schizophrenia. *Archives of General Psychiatry, 43,* 633–642.

Kohlenberg, R. J., & Tsai, M. (1991). *Functional analytic psychotherapy: Creating intense and curative therapeutic relationships.* New York: Plenum Press.

Kutchins, H., & Kirk, S. A. (1986). The reliability of DSM-III: A critical review. *Social Work Research & Abstracts, 22*(4), 3–12.

Link, B. (1987). Understanding labeling effects in mental disorders: An assessment of expectations of rejection. *American Sociological Review, 52,* 96–112.

Lowery, C. T. (in press). *Reclaiming the spirit: The addiction and recovery of Native American women.* Madison: University of Wisconsin Press.

Mattaini, M. A. (1994). Can personalities be disordered? No! In S. A. Kirk & S. Einbinder (Eds.), *Controversial issues in mental health* (pp. 48–56). Needham Heights, MA: Allyn & Bacon.

Mattaini, M. A., & Kirk, S. A. (1991). Assessing assessment in social work. *Social Work, 36,* 260–266.

McLaughlin, M., & Pepper, B. (1990). The young and the restless: Programming for the crisis-ridden young adult patient. In N. L. Cohen (Ed.), *Psychiatry takes to the streets* (pp. 137–155). New York: Guilford Press.

Mischel, W. (1968). *Personality and assessment.* New York: John Wiley & Sons.

Mischel, W. (1986). *Introduction to personality: A new look* (4th ed.). New York: Holt, Rinehart & Winston.

Patterson, G. R. (1976). The aggressive child: Victim and architect of a coercive system. In E. J. Mash, L. A. Hamerlynck, & L. C. Handy (Eds.), *Behavior modification and families* (pp. 267–316). New York: Brunner/Mazel.

Reid, W. J. (1992). *Task strategies.* New York: Columbia University Press.

Rossi, P. (1989). *Down and out in America: The origins of homelessness.* Chicago: University of Chicago Press.

Wallace, C. J., & Liberman, R. P. (1985). Social skills training of patients with schizophrenia: A controlled clinical trial. *Psychiatry Research, 15,* 239–247.

Wong, S. E. (1996). Psychosis. In M. A. Mattaini & B. A. Thyer (Eds.), *Finding solutions to social problems: Behavioral strategies for change* (pp. 319–343). Washington, DC: APA Books.

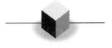

INDEX

behavioral ecomaps for, 18–19,
34–35, 39
behaviorally anchored rating
scale, 34
of client behavior in session,
27–28
of client goals, 32
client–social worker relationship
in, 22
contingency diagrams, 42
data sources, 33, 34, 35, 36–37
of depression and demoralization, 98–99
diagnostic labeling, 45–46
ecobehavioral approach, xii,
29–32
ecobehavioral scan, 33–38
equivalence relations problems,
65
goals, 28, 46–47, 96–97
intervention design, 44–45
monitoring case progress, 39
motivational interviewing,
143–145
nonlinear approach, 29
organic etiology, 46
person-in-environment system,
46
for problem drinking, 156–157
of problem solving skills, 57
self-monitoring data, 33, 34, 74,
75, 77
setting clinical goals, 38–40
setting for, 91
significance of, 22
standardized instruments, 36–38

of suicidality, 99–102
time allocated for, 22
Automatic thoughts, 61

B

Behavioral contingencies
assessment, 40–44
clinical significance, xiii, 17
definition and characteristics,
15–16
diagrams of, 42
matching law, 16
natural, 4
rule-governed behavior and, 13
Behavioral theory
antecedent determinants of
behavior, 8–11
concept of self, 15
consequences as determinants of
behavior, 2–8, 13
contingencies, 15–17
determinants of behavior,
1–2
in ecobehavioral approach, 17
emotions in, 12–13
equivalence relations in, 14
rate determinants, 8–9
respondent behavior, 15
rule-governed behavior, 13–14
scope, 2
significance of private experiences, 11–12
for social work practice, ix
terminology, 1
Brief interventions, xi

C

Clinical Practice with Individuals

self-talk patterns, 104–105
therapeutic relationship, 104
Deprivation, 10
Desensitization interventions, 114
Diagnostic and Statistical Manual of Mental Disorders, 46
depressive disorders, 98
Diagnostic classification, 45–46
personality disorders, 167, 179
Differential reinforcement, 4–5
of incompatible behavior, 5
of other behavior, 5
of rates of behavior, 5
Discriminative stimuli, 9
Duration of intervention, xi

E

Ecobehavioral practice
applications, xiii
assessment, xii, 29–32
characteristics, x–xi
client resource issues, xiii
clinical goals, 17–18
cognitive components, 56
concept of pathology, 15, 19
concept of self in, 15
conception of self-talk, 12
conceptual basis, 1, 17, 19
duration of intervention, xi
empowerment in, 115
goals, xi–xii, 91
hopeful perspective of, 20
implementation, xi
maintaining change in, xii, 17
settings for, 90–92

significance of behavioral contingencies, 15
strategic nature, 47
terminology, 1
Ecobehavioral scan, 33–38
addiction assessment, 149–150
Ecomaps, 18–19, 34–35
for assessing depression, 102
for monitoring case progress, 39
Emotion
acceptance of, 67–69, 113–114
behavioral perspective, 12–13
expressed, in families of mentally ill clients, 175
expressing feelings, 126–127
inoculation training for coping, 86–88
self-talk processes, 60–61
as target of interventions, 98
Empowerment
clinical significance, 115
through intervention planning, 49
through pharmacotherapy, 106–107
through self-monitoring, 74
Equivalence relations, 14
about mental illness, 171
clinical use, 24
depression intervention, 112–113
in mental illness, 180
patterns in depression, 105
persistence of, 112
as self-talk problem, 65–66
self-talk problems, 61

Exercise, 76
Experimenting with life, 51–52,
    54–55
    alternative relationship behav-
        iors, 135–136
    social network support, 137–138
    treating depression, 114–119
Exposure therapies, 69–71

F

Families
    in addiction treatment process,
        152–155
    embedding new practices, 49–50
    influence on addictive behaviors,
        151–152
    intervention with mentally ill
        client, 175–176
Feedback, for relationship skills
    training, 132
Fixed-role therapy, 52–53
Flooding, 70

G

Gestalt therapy, 56

H

Home sessions/tasks
    advantages, 91, 92–93
    disadvantages, 91
    ecobehavioral approach, 91–92
    monitoring, 92, 93
    for relationship skills training,
        132–133

relaxation exercises for, 88
techniques, 93

I

Imaging techniques, 83
Imitation, 11
Incentives and rewards, 2–3
Individual practice, x, 120
Inoculation techniques, 71, 86–88
Interpersonal psychotherapy,
    116–117
Interpersonal relations
    accepting/providing feedback,
        128
    aggression/violence in, 135,
        138–140
    appropriate use of relationship
        skills, 133–136
    being nonprovocable, 129
    cause of depression, 103–104
    clinical goals, 122–124
    community reinforcement
        approach, 161
    conversational skills, 127–128
    cultural considerations, 120–122,
        134–135
    depression interventions,
        116–118
    embedding new practices,
        49–51
    experimentation, 51–52
    expressing feelings, 126–127
    expressing opinions, 127
    individual work for, 120
    learning repertoires for, 124
    listening skills, 125–126

making refusals, 129

making requests for behavior change, 128–129

negotiating skills, 129–130

patterns of addiction and, 151–152

personal disclosure in, 127

positive reinforcement effects, 4

practicing alternative behaviors, 135–136

showing empathy, 126

skills training for mentally ill client, 173–174

social network support skills, 136–138

social reinforcers for, 124–125

techniques for skills training, 130–133

Interventive techniques

acceptance and commitment therapy, 56, 57, 67–69

addiction treatment, 152–155

with aggressive/violent behavior, 135

with ambivalent client, 60

appropriate use of relationship skills, 133–136

behavioral shaping, 5

choices and consequences strategy, 57–60

for client with mental illness, 169–181

cognitive strategies, 45, 56–57

community reinforcement approach, 158–165

consideration of structural factors, 10–11

for depression and demoralization, 98, 105–118

differential reinforcement, 4–5

embedding new experiences/ practices, 49–51

empowerment through, 49

experimenting with life, 51–52

exposure, 69–71

fixed-role therapy, 52–53

learning relationship repertoires, 130–133

for maintaining change, 94–97

matching law theory, 15

modeling for imitation, 11

motivating antecedents, 9–10

for negative self-talk, 28, 60–66

nonreinforcement, 6

paradoxical, 66

pharmacotherapy, 106–107

positive reinforcement, 3–4

for problem drinking, 155–157

punishment, 6–8

for respondent behaviors, 15

self-management, 75–79

self-monitoring, 74

skills training, 73–74

strategic use, 47

for supporting social network, 136–138

task planning and implementation sequence, 54–55

treatment planning, 44

types of, 47

for violent relationships, 140

equivalence relations in, 180
family systems work, 175–176
lifestyle enrichment, 176–177
pharmacotherapy for, 169–170
psychoeducation for, 170–171
self-experience in, 179–180
social work counseling goals, 167–168
symptom management, 171–173
young adult chronic clients, 177–181
See also specific disorders
Punishment
clinical use, 6–8
definition, 6
intergenerational transmission, 7
versus negative reinforcement, 1, 5

R

Rational disputation, 62–63
depression intervention, 109–110
Rational-emotive therapy, 56
Rehearsal of relationship skills, 130–131
Reinforcer sampling, 10, 115–116
Relapse prevention, 149–150
Relaxation exercises, 70–71
application, 79, 85
breathing techniques, 81
home sessions, 88
for immediate coping, 80
interrupting negative self-talk, 83–85
muscle relaxation techniques, 81–83

practicing, 79–80
for reducing cumulative stress, 80
techniques, 80–81, 85–86
visualization techniques, 83
Respondent behavior, 15
Respondent conditioning, 13
Risk-taking, for decreasing excessive rule governance, 64–65
Role playing, 52–53
Rule-governed behavior, 13–14
excessive, 64–65
self-talk problems, 60, 61
Rules, 12
definition, 13
depressive self-talk, 109
inaccurate, as self-talk, 61–62

S

Schedule of reinforcement, 3–4
for maintaining clinical change, 94–95
Schemas, self-talk as, 61–62
Schizophrenia, 167, 169–170
Self
cultural concepts, 121
ecobehavioral conceptualization, 15
experience in mental illness, 179–180
Self-instructional training, 86
Self-management, 14, 60
design of objectives, 76–77
focus on consequences, 77–78
goal setting, 76
monitoring compliance, 77
reinforcement, 78–79

requirements for, 76, 79

Self-monitoring, 33, 60

  in addiction intervention, 147–148

  applications, 75

  for changing equivalence relations, 66

  for changing inaccurate rules, 64

  of home tasks, 92, 93

  as intervention, 74, 92

Self-talk

  clinical conceptualizations, 12

  clinical goals, 28

  collaborative empiricism for, 63

  decreasing excessive rule governance, 64–65

  in depression, 104–105

  emotional processing, 60–61

  equivalence relations problems, 65–66

  for examination of delusional thinking, 172–173

  exposure interventions with, 69–70

  of inaccurate rules, 61–62

  inoculation technique, 86

  interventions for depression, 108–113

  interventive strategies, 61–66

  practice log, 64

  rational disputation of, 62–63

  for relationship skills training, 132

  relaxation techniques for interrupting, 83–85

  rules as, 13

Shaping, behavioral, 5

Skills training

  appropriate use of relationship skills, 133–136

  for client with mental illness, 173–174

  for community reinforcement approach, 163

  contingent feedback, 132

  inoculation techniques, 86–88

  learning relationship repertoires, 130–133

  in natural environment, 92–93

  relationship repertoires, 124–130

  relaxation techniques, 79–86

  for social network support, 136–138

  techniques, 73–74

  transfer to natural environment, 93–94

Social learning, 11

Social reinforcement, 50–51

  addictive behaviors, 149

  cultural considerations, 125

  in etiology of depression, 102–103, 104

  learning, 123–125

  for maintaining change, 96

  network support skills, 136–137

  in treating depression, 116–118

Social work practice, goals of, ix–x

Sociocultural considerations

  in community reinforcement approach, 164–165

  listening behavior, 126

  relationship issues, 121–122, 134–135

  social reinforcement, 125

ABOUT THE AUTHOR

Mark A. Mattaini, DSW, ACSW, is associate professor, Columbia University School of Social Work; chair, Walden Fellowship, Inc.; and director, Musher Seminar Series on Science and Human Behavior, Columbia University, and holds the NASW Diplomate in Clinical Practice. His current research deals with applications of the science of behavior to serious social problems including youth violence and child maltreatment. His previous books include *More Than a Thousand Words: Graphics for Clinical Practice* (NASW Press, 1993); *The Foundations of Social Work Practice: A Graduate Text* (with Carol H. Meyer) (NASW Press, 1995); and *Finding Solutions to Social Problems: Behavioral Strategies for Change* (with Bruce A. Thyer) (American Psychological Association, 1996). Dr. Mattaini also does clinical and community practice in New York City.

Clinical Practice with Individuals

Designed by Naylor Design, Inc.

Composed by Toni L. Milbourne and Patricia D. Wolf, Wolf Publications, Inc., in Jenson and Myriad.

Printed by Automated Graphics Systems on 60# Williamsburg Offset Smooth.

PRACTICE RESOURCES FOR SOCIAL WORKERS

Clinical Practice with Individuals, *by Mark A. Mattaini.* Practitioners and educators alike will find this guidebook invaluable. Mattaini presents practice guidelines that are firmly rooted in contemporary state-of-the-art knowledge and both accessible and immediately applicable to practice.
ISBN: 0-87101-270-7. Item #2707. Price $28.95

Person-in-Environment System: The PIE Classification System, *James M. Karls and Karin E. Wandrei, Editors.* Demonstrates how to use PIE to facilitate social work practice. Helps clinicians better understand their clients. A valuable teaching tool for social work practice courses. Used by administrators to develop agency and community programs. Also available in a set with the *PIE Manual.*
ISBN: 0-87101-240-5. Item #2405A. Price $28.95

PIE Manual, *James M. Karls and Karin E. Wandrei, Editors.* Lists the descriptions, classifications, and codes used in PIE and includes case examples to help familiarize readers with the PIE system. Also available in a set with the *Person-in-Environment System.*
ISBN: 0-87101-254-5. Item #2545. Price $28.95

Person-in-Environment System (2-volume set). When purchased together, the *Person-in-Environment System* and *PIE Manual* serve as a major tool for classifying and codifying problems in social functioning. Applications are useful for social work practitioners, students, administrators, researchers, and educators, as well as social policymakers and community organizers.
Item #2405. Price $38.95

Managed Care Resource Guides, *Vivian H. Jackson, Editor.* These guides provide essential information to help practitioners advance social work within a managed care environment. Each guide contains an overview of the issues and information on the knowledge and skills necessary for effective practice in a specialized environment.
Agency Settings: ISBN: 0-87101-245-6. Item #2456. Price $50
Private Practice: ISBN: 0-87101-247-2. Item #2472. Price $50

(Order form on reverse side)

ORDER FORM

Title	Item #	Price	Total
__ Clinical Practice with Individuals	Item 2707	$28.95	_____
__ Person-in-Environment System Book	Item 2405A	$28.95	_____
__ Person-in-Environment System Manual	Item 2545	$28.95	_____
__ Person-in-Environment System (book and manual)	Item 2405	$38.95	_____
__ Managed Care Resource Guide— Agency Setting	Item 2456	$50.00	_____
__ Managed Care Resource Guide— Private Practice	Item 2472	$50.00	_____
		Subtotal	_____
	+ 10% postage and handling		_____
		Total	_____

❒ I've enclosed my check or money order for $ _____.

❒ Please charge my   ❒ NASW Visa*   ❒ Other Visa   ❒ MasterCard

_____   _____
Credit Card Number   Expiration Date

Signature _____

Use of this card generates funds in support of the social work profession.

Name_____

Address _____

City _____ State/Province _____

Country _____ Zip _____

Phone _____   _____
                                              NASW Member # (if applicable)

(Please make checks payable to NASW Press. Prices are subject to change.)

NASW PRESS

NASW Press
P.O. Box 431
Annapolis JCT, MD 20701
USA

Credit card orders call
1-800-227-3590
(In the Metro Wash., DC, area, call 301-317-8688)
Or fax your order to 301-206-7989
Or e-mail nasw@pmds.com

Visit our Web site at http://www.naswpress.org   CPWIBI96